Who Cares?

DATE			

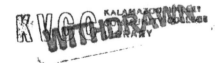
BAKER & TAYLOR

WHO CARES?

Institutional Barriers to Health Care for Lesbian, Gay, and Bisexual Persons

Michele J. Eliason, PhD, RN

NLN Press • New York

Pub. No. 14-6762

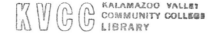

Copyright © 1996
National League for Nursing
350 Hudson Street, New York, NY 10014

The views expressed in this book reflect those of the authors and do not necessarily reflect the official views of the National League for Nursing.

Library of Congress Cataloging-in-Publication Data

Eliason, Michele J.
    Who Cares? : institutional barriers to health care for lesbian,
gay, and bisexual persons / Michele J. Eliason.
        p.   cm.
    Includes bibliographical references and index.
    ISBN 0-88737-676-2
    1. Gays—Medical care.   2. Bisexuals—Medical care.
3. Discrimination in medical care.   4. Medical personnel—Attitudes.
5. Homophobia.   I. Title.
RA564.9.H65E45   1996
362.1'08'664—dc20   96-17319
                                                                                              CIP

This book was set in Garamond by Publications Development Company, Crockett, Texas. The editor and designer was Allan Graubard. The printer was Book Crafters. The cover was designed by Lauren Stevens.

Printed in the United States of America.

Acknowledgments

Writing this book has been an enlightening experience. I learned how little we actually know about lesbian, gay, and bisexual health care, yet I was encouraged to discover that the number of articles and books about these issues has increased in the past few years. I was appalled to find many examples of unscientific thinking and bigoted conjecture in the health care literature, yet I was also happy to find many pleas for compassion and acceptance. The varied responses to this project were intriguing. Some people asked me if writing such a book as a junior faculty member was wise, implying that the subject was "too risky." Yet others suggested that they did not think of this work as part of my academic career, but as some odd hobby or personal agenda. Still others asked what I was working on, and when I told them the title of the book, they simply replied, "Oh," and seemed embarrassed.

I wrote much of this book at a table in a local deli/bakery (if you are ever in Iowa City, I can highly recommend *The Cottage*) and often encountered colleagues, friends, and acquaintances there. When they would ask what I was working on, many of them seemed uncomfortable if I said "lesbian, gay, and bisexual" in a normal voice. They looked around to see if other customers had heard, or stepped back as if to distance themselves from me. Sometimes, strangers at the next table would look furtively at the titles of the books and articles spread out before me. They seemed surprised that I didn't try to hide these titles. One person even moved to a table on the other side of the restaurant. These experiences reaffirmed the need for this book. It is time to discuss these issues openly.

Many people were instrumental in the completion of this book: My parents, who always encouraged me to do what I thought was right, and continue to support me in all I do; my siblings and their families, who also support and nurture me; the lesbian, gay, and bisexual community in my hometown, who sustained me through my own coming out process; my academic colleagues, especially those in the University of Iowa Lesbian, Gay, and Bisexual Staff and Faculty Association, who encouraged me to study lesbian, gay, and bisexual health care issues; and those brave few researchers, who first broke the silence on these topics at great personal risk.

I also want to thank the NLN Press first, for recognizing the need for and soliciting material on lesbian, gay, and bisexual health, and second, for supporting and publishing my work. Thanks especially to Allan Graubard for his encouragement and helpful suggestions.

Finally, I want to dedicate the book to my life partner, Obiagele. Her love sustains me in all that I do.

About the Author

Michele J. Eliason, PhD, RN, is an assistant professor in the College of Nursing at the University of Iowa. She is trained as both a psychologist and a nurse. Dr. Eliason's research in the past eight years has focused on attitudes toward lesbian, gay, and bisexual people, and in particular, attitudes of nurses; sexual identity development; and physical and mental health issues for lesbian, gay, and bisexual people.

Contents

1 Introduction   **1**

Two Philosophies   3
Prejudice   5
Sharon and Karen's Story   7
How Many Lesbian, Gay, and Bisexual People
   Are There?   10
Organization of This Book   13
EXERCISE: Determining Your Own Sexual
   Identity   14

2 Lesbian, Gay, and Bisexual Issues   **17**

Historical Overview   18
Basic Terminology   24
   Homophobia   27
   Internalized Homophobia   32
   Heterosexism   33
Coming Out   37
Diversity in Lesbian, Gay, and Bisexual Communities   45
   Racial and Ethnic Diversity   45
   Gender   51
   Class   52
   Age   53
   Religion   53
   Political Involvement   54
Origins or "Causes" of Sexual Orientation   55
   Biologically Based Theories   56
   Environmental Theories   58

Conclusion   59
EXERCISE: Am I Homophobic?   59

3   The Damage Done by Negative Stereotypes   **62**

Doesn't the Bible Condemn Homosexuality?   63
Aren't Homosexuals Confused about Their
    Sex or Gender?   67
Homosexuality Is Caused by a Bad Experience with
    the Opposite Sex   69
Isn't There a Link between Homosexuality and
    Child Molestation?   70
Homosexual Relationships Don't Last   71
Aren't Homosexuals Obsessed with Sex?   72
Lesbian, Gay, and Bisexual People "Flaunt"
    Their Sexuality   73
Homosexuals Could Change Their Preference
    If They Tried   75
Didn't Homosexuals Bring AIDS to the
    United States?   77
Aren't Bisexuals Just Confused about
    Their Identities?   78
Conclusion   80
EXERCISE: Exploring Stereotypes   80

4   Lesbian, Gay, and Bisexual Family Issues   **81**

Family of Origin Issues   83
Gay and Lesbian Couples as Chosen Family   87
    Social Support for Same-Sex Couples   87
    Same-Sex Couple Relationship
       Characteristics   88
    Relationship Satisfaction and Sources
       of Conflict   89
    Disclosure of Sexual Identity to Health
       Care Providers   91
    Violence and Same-Sex Couples   92
    Living with Illness or Disability   94
    Hospitalization   95
Lesbian, Gay, and Bisexual Families with Children   95
    Issues That May Affect Children   95
    Coming Out to Children   100
    Unique Problems with Children   102

Strategies for Health Care Providers   103
EXERCISE: "Family Values"   105

5   Health Care Provider Attitudes   **107**

Attitudes of Health Care Providers   109
    Surveys of Health Care Providers about
      Their Attitudes   112
    Attitudes about AIDS and Homosexuality:
      A Deadly Interaction   117
Experiences of Lesbian, Gay, and Bisexual People with
  Health Care Providers   119
    Disclosure of Sexual Identity to Health
      Care Providers   119
    Lesbian, Gay, and Bisexual People's Perceptions
      of Their Health Care   121
Potential Behavioral Consequences of
  Negative Attitudes   128
Conclusion   129
EXERCISE: Predictors of Negative Attitudes   129

6   Sexual Identity and Developmental Transitions   **131**

Childhood   131
Adolescence   139
    Coming Out   142
    Depression and Suicide   143
    Violence, Homelessness, and Prostitution   143
    Sexually Transmitted Infections, HIV,
      and Pregnancy   144
    Guidelines for Working with Lesbian, Gay, and
      Bisexual Teens   145
    Working with Parents of Lesbian, Gay, and
      Bisexual Teens   146
Young Adulthood   147
    Coming Out   148
    Forming Intimate Relationships   149
    Commitment to a Partner and Beginning
      a Family   150
    Career and Work Issues   150
Middle Adulthood   151

Reproductive Transitions: Menopause   153
Men at Midlife   154
Older Adulthood   155
  Elder Services and Lesbian, Gay, and
    Bisexual People   158
  EXERCISE: Planning for Our Old Age   160

7   Lesbian and Bisexual Women's Health   **161**

Lesbian and Bisexual Women's Physical Health   163
  Regular Gynecological Care   164
  Sexually Transmitted Infections Other
    Than HIV   166
  HIV/AIDS   166
  Cancers   170
  Sexual Dysfunctions   171
  Pregnancy-Related Issues   172
Lesbian and Bisexual Women's Mental Health   173
  Substance Abuse and Misuse   175
  Depression and Suicide   181
  Eating Disorders   182
  Hate Crimes   183
Interviewing Lesbian and Bisexual Female
  Clients or Patients   184
Conclusion   186
EXERCISE: Is Your Own Organization Inclusive?   187

8   Gay and Bisexual Men's Health   **188**

Gay and Bisexual Men's Mental Health   189
  Hate Crimes   189
  Potential Consequences of Internalized
    Homophobia   192
Gay and Bisexual Men's Physical Health   200
  Unsafe Sexual Experiences   200
  HIV/AIDS   203
  Health Care Provider Attitudes about AIDS   204
  Prevention of HIV   207
Conclusion   209
EXERCISE: AIDS in Real Life   210

9   Making Health Care Safe and Inclusive   **211**

Society and the Healthy Homosexual   212
Health Care Institutions   214
        Education and Training   216
        Policies and Procedures   220
Individual Health Care Providers   225
Conclusion   229
EXERCISE: A Glimpse of Lesbian, Gay, or
Bisexual Life   230

10   Afterword   **231**

Appendix: Sample Durable Power of Attorney
        for Health Care   **235**

References   **239**

Index   **265**

CHAPTER ONE

Introduction

As I WRITE THIS COLUMN, I am lying in a hospital bed in the cardiac care unit of a Philadelphia hospital a short ambulance ride from my house. It is 1 A.M. and the unit is eerily quiet except for the constant beeping of heart monitors, like the one to which I am hooked up, and the whoosh and whir of machines that automatically inflate blood pressure cuffs on the arms of patients. There is an oxygen tube in my nose and an IV line in my arm, the colorless air and the equally colorless fluid make no sound as they help restore the balance of my body's chemistry.

This eerie night seems a fitting end to a terrifying day. It began in the most mundane of places: the shower. My heart began to beat very fast and very oddly, turning over in my chest, as if the top and bottom halves of my heart were on separate paths, bound for collision. By the time I lay down on my bed, my wet hair streaming down my back, I felt as if I were suffocating, gasping for air as my heart twisted and beat through my chest like an Edgar Allen Poe heart.

It took only five minutes for the rescue squad to arrive. As my partner, Judith, led them upstairs to our bedroom, I had a wave of thinking that she shouldn't have called 911, that this oddity would pass, that I would be fine. But an EKG and IV later, I was watching my neighborhood rush past the blurred windows of the ambulance on my way to the ER with my atrially fibrillating heart.

I don't think about being a lesbian much—not actively, at least. I rarely think about it outside of the context of activism or appearing on someone's radio program or television talk show. It's intrinsic, like being blond or blue-eyed or tall.

But I become acutely aware of my lesbianism in certain circumstances. And it's the first thing I think about when I enter a

1

*hospital. I think about the questions I will be asked and the an-
swers I will give. I will, for example, be asked about my next of
kin. If I were straight, that would be Judith. But when I say, "Judith," I am invariably asked if she is my sister. "No," I say, "we
live together." They tell me that if she is not related, she is my
friend, not my next of kin. I give them the name and number of
my married sister. Then I am asked when my last period was
and if I could be pregnant. I say "no" and am asked if I am
"sure." "Yes," I say, "I am positive." I ask if pregnancy causes
atrial fibrillation and the doctor looks confused. He doesn't ask
again if I am pregnant.*

    *I want to know two things: if I am going to die and if Judith
can stay with me in the ER while I wait for a bed to become
available in the cardiac care unit in intensive care, in the part
of the hospital that is most frightening because it is closest to
death. In spite of the pregnancy harangue, this doctor is very
nice; he tells me that Judith can stay.*

    *. . . There is no question: I'm scared, I don't want Judith to
leave, I don't want to be alone in the ER or the CCU, once I get
there. No one knows why my heart is beating the way it is; no
one can tell me when the drug will begin to work. And in the
midst of my sickening fear, I have to worry: worry that she is
only my "friend"—not my wife, my husband, my fiancee—not
my "real" kin, even after seven years, a mortgage, a car, six cats,
a dog and a shared business.*

    *This is what equal rights for queers comes down to: whether
or not my partner can stay with me in the hospital just like her
father's wife stayed with him when he was in a cardiac care
unit a year ago. It seems so very basic: You're sick and frightened, you might die and the person who is most important to
you in the world becomes a cipher, someone who doesn't fit into
the heterosexual hierarchy of importance.*

    *I am fortunate—out of the closet and brave enough to tell the
cardiologist that Judith is my partner, that I want her to stay
with me, that I have a right to have her with me. But what
about all the queers who can't fight hospital hierarchies or who
fear disclosure because homophobia is so oppressive? These
women and men suffer—and sometimes die—alone. In the
greenish glow of the CCU, I am still scared. But sleeping in a
chair a few feet from me is Judith—close enough to touch, close
enough to hear my whispered, "I love you," close enough to keep
my fear at bay.*

> *Would straight America lose so much if lesbians and gay men*
> *were allowed such basic rights, too? Could compassion really be*
> *that costly? (Victoria Brownworth, 1995, p. 50, reprinted with*
> *permission of* Deneuve Magazine*)*

Brownworth's column reflects many of the fears of lesbian, gay, and bisexual people who must be hospitalized; fears that too much of the time are based on reality. What would it take to grant her wish—to extend compassion and basic human rights to lesbian, gay, and bisexual people? This book will address health care issues for lesbian, gay, and bisexual people, and in particular, the attitudes of health care providers, the potential effects of these attitudes on lesbian, gay, and bisexual patients/clients and their partners, and the institutional policies that can discriminate against some patients and clients.

TWO PHILOSOPHIES

Our Western society is in turmoil over the changes in demography, family structures and values, and provision of health care. As the United States becomes more visibly multicultural and as culturally diverse people challenge traditional values and philosophies, growth is likely. But along with growth comes considerable conflict, anxieties, and fears about change. People who differ from the norm in terms of race or sexual identity threaten to disrupt the comfortable status quo and force white, heterosexual people to face their prejudices and fears. Although the issues of race and sexuality in contemporary society are not identical, there are many similarities and points of overlap and intersection. For example, stereotypes about African Americans include the idea that they are "oversexed" or more primitive in their sexual practices (West, 1993). Stereotypes about lesbian, gay, and bisexual people similarly focus on sexual excesses and promiscuity (Blumenfeld & Raymond, 1988; Eliason, Donelan, & Randall, 1992).

Some lesbian, gay, and bisexual people are also Asian American, Native American, Latino, or African American, resulting in experiences of multiple oppressions. For example, the Latina lesbian may be oppressed because of her ethnicity, gender, and sexuality (and woe unto her if she is older as well). Yet some people in our society believe that only white people can be lesbian, gay, or bisexual, further rendering gay people of color invisible. There is growing evidence that prejudice is often a global phenomenon, so that the person who has negative attitudes about a particular racial group is likely also to have negative attitudes about lesbian, gay, and bisexual people (Bierly, 1985; Ficarrotto, 1990). All of us are socialized into a culture that is inherently racist, sexist, and homophobic, and we all learn the stereotypes and negative attitudes to some extent. How do health care systems currently address these negative attitudes? Does health care education attempt to reduce prejudice in any way? How do the negative attitudes of health care providers affect patient care?

The most commonly cited philosophy found in all the health care professions (and in U.S. society in general) concerns equal treatment: that is, we treat all patients/clients the same regardless of any human characteristic such as race, sex, ethnicity, religion, or ability to pay. This attitude permeates health care ideology and is often employed to explain why we don't need specific course work on cultural diversity or women's health. If we treat everyone exactly the same, then there is no need to learn about individual differences. This argument is also employed in society as a whole to argue against affirmative action or scholarships based on race, and to argue against civil rights laws to protect lesbian, gay, and bisexual people from harassment and discrimination. Equal treatment simply makes race, gender, or sexuality irrelevant. However, people are *not* treated equally in our society or in health care. Prejudices, fears, and negative attitudes are so deeply ingrained in individuals and in institutions that discrimination is widespread. Equally significant is its commonality, its *routine* character, which makes it largely invisible to those in the dominant group. One only need to glance at the statistics, however, to measure its effects: people of color are more likely to receive substandard or no health care at all (White, 1990); women have been neglected by medical research (Oakley, 1993); and lesbian, gay, and bisexual people have been mistreated, even harassed, by health care providers (Cotton, 1992; Stevens & Hall, 1988). In this light, equal treatment becomes a vague philosophy at best, whose potential in practice remains to be seen. And if, all of a sudden, we did treat everyone equally, would that improve health outcomes? Probably not. Equal treatment, which assumes that one kind of treatment is best for all people, fails to account for the numerous mediating variables affecting health outcomes, which we have only recently, and painfully, become aware of. Wouldn't it be better to take these into account from the beginning?

One alternative here involves adopting a culturally relevant philosophy and model of health care, beginning with this assumption: all people deserve *equal access* to health care, but may require different assessment and treatment options for specific individual needs—with a likely result in better health care outcomes for patients/clients and their families. At the same time, such attention to individual needs may also require a major shift in health care educational programs and health care delivery systems. Learning culturally sensitive health care assessment methods and practices while unlearning prejudices becomes paramount. But this, too, is easier said than done. Prejudices are as deeply ingrained in individuals as they are in health care systems. In this book, then, I will explore some of the ways that prejudices have become institutionalized and will offer some solutions for reducing prejudice at both the individual and institutional levels.

Prejudice

What is a prejudice? A prejudice is: (1) a preconceived, usually unfavorable idea; (2) an opinion held in disregard of facts that contradict it; a bias; (3) intolerance or hatred of other races; (4) injury or harm (*Webster's New World Dictionary,* 1987). Prejudice about people who differ from us by race or ethnicity is called *racism;* prejudice against women is called *sexism;* and prejudice against lesbian, gay, or bisexual people is called *homophobia* or *heterosexism* (terms to be explained in detail in Chapter 2). Unlearning prejudice still presents many difficulties. Prejudicial attitudes are absorbed by the young long before they can understand them. By the time understanding occurs, ideas about groups of people, which often carry strong emotional connotations, are already deeply ingrained. For example, children can learn negative messages about lesbian, gay, and bisexual people via:

- Taunts of "fag" and "queer" and "sissy" on the playground—young children often do not know what the words mean, but they know they are really bad.
- Antigay jokes told by friends, siblings, parents.
- Friends, siblings, or parents who laugh at antigay jokes.
- The absence of positive gay role models in their schools, churches, scout troops, athletic teams, and so on.

- Explicit antigay teaching in some churches and by some parents and teachers.
- Subtle reactions of parents, such as turning off the TV when gay people are mentioned, avoiding gay neighbors, refusing to discuss or omitting homosexuality from discussions of sex education.
- Antigay graffiti on bathroom walls or public areas.
- TV sitcoms that use gay characters for the punch line.
- Antigay song lyrics or comments in movies, concerts, etc.
- A family's big secret—a lesbian, gay, or bisexual family member whom they whisper about or avoid discussing around the children.
- School boards that prohibit discussion of homosexuality in school-based sex education programs.
- Local community groups that burn or ban gay-positive children's books such as *Heather Has Two Mommies.*

Everyone has some degree of prejudice about some group of people. Some people are racist, others hate people who are overweight, some don't trust disabled people, others dislike Catholics, Jews, or Muslims, and so on. We cannot have a variety of direct experiences, or obtain formal learning about all possible types of people. Prejudices are based on limited or inaccurate information, lack of direct experience, or on a few, isolated negative experiences. The danger of prejudice, though, is that it assumes that all people of a particular group are alike and have the same negative qualities. In effect, prejudice takes the humanity away from people. When considering health care delivery, it is crucial, then, to explore how prejudice is expressed, and whether it will affect the quality of health care an individual obtains. In a later chapter, I will consider the ways that prejudice against lesbian, gay, and bisexual people might manifest in health care providers' actions. But one fact is clear from social psychological research—there is no direct one-to-one relationship between attitudes and behavior (Festinger, 1964; Triandis, 1982; Wicker, 1969). Some people have very negative attitudes, but do not actively harass or discriminate against people of that group. Others are accepting of diverse people, but stand by and allow discrimination to occur for fear of intervening or of being labeled as a member of that group. In general, however, the more negative the attitude is, the more likely it will be expressed in the person's behavior. We are also learning that prejudice is unhealthy, both for the group targeted by such thinking, and for the person who reacts with prejudice. Prejudice creates fear and discomfort in social relationships and limits the social network of the individual. Prejudice can disrupt friendships, break apart families, and even start wars (Blumenfeld, 1992).

To round out this somewhat abstract discussion of prejudice, stop now for a moment and imagine this situation: Your significant other, a person you love deeply and with whom you plan to spend the rest of your life, has been critically injured in a car accident. How would you feel? Probably you would experience some degree of panic, fear, overwhelming anxiety, maybe anger, perhaps a physical pain in your gut. Keep these feelings in mind while you read the following true story.

SHARON AND KAREN'S STORY

In November 1983, Sharon Kowalski left the home she shared with her lover, Karen Thompson, to drive her niece and nephew home to Northern Minnesota. Their car was struck by a drunken driver, killing the niece and seriously injuring the nephew and Sharon. Karen, who had been her significant other for four years, rushed to the hospital but could not see Sharon nor receive information about her condition because she was not "immediate family." Later she discovered that Sharon had sustained a severe head injury and was in a coma. When Karen was finally allowed to see her, this was her reaction:

> *I didn't know what to expect. Will she remember me? I wondered. Will she remember our relationship? She might wake up at any minute and ask for me. How will that look? Will people guess about our relationship? Still not comprehending the full extent of Sharon's injuries, I feared for our own secrecy as much as I feared for her life. (Thompson & Andrzejewski, 1988, pp. 5-6)*

Why the fear? Because Karen and Sharon had led a secret life together. Although they had made a commitment to each other and had exchanged rings, they had not told any family members about their relationship and had revealed it to only a few close friends. Only recently had Sharon stated that she was gay—before they had only talked about their personal situation and had not related it to their own sexual orientations. They had not really thought of themselves as a lesbian couple as much as they considered themselves two people in love, who happened to be women. After the accident, Karen spent as much time as possible with Sharon. As a physical education teacher, she knew something about the importance of rehabilitation and began assisting the hospital staff with range of motion and other activities. During those first few awful months, Sharon's parents who lived three hours away, often stayed at the home Karen and Sharon had shared:

> *It was during one of those stays that the Kowalskis must have found something that indicated the true nature of Sharon's and my relationship. They moved out of the house without telling me. That evening at the hospital, Donald Kowalski asked me to leave the room and talk with him in the hall. He stated that no one could love Sharon like family could love Sharon. He said that the family could meet all of her needs; that friends weren't supposed to visit as often as I was visiting and if I didn't stop visiting so often, he would see to it I couldn't visit at all. (Thompson & Andrzejewski, 1988, p. 17)*

Since the parents were not able to visit daily and therefore could not monitor Karen's visits, she continued her vigil at Sharon's side, but in fear that each visit might be her last. Sharon began the slow process of recovery with minimal voluntary movement and increasing periods of alertness. Although Karen continued to care for her and talk to her about the future, she was agonizing about the reaction of Sharon's parents to their true relationship and began to talk with a psychologist about revealing it. They decided that a letter would be the best method of approach. In January 1984, Karen sent a letter explaining how much she loved Sharon, that she and Sharon had planned a future together, and that she needed to be centrally involved in Sharon's recovery. The Kowalski family reacted in anger, denying that their daughter could be a lesbian. Karen was in turmoil; her significant other was permanently disabled and in need of considerable support and she feared the Kowalskis would attempt to cut her out of Sharon's life. While going through this trauma, she also had to deal directly with her own sexuality. This latter process involved reconciling her strong, conservative religious beliefs with what she knew about her relationship with Sharon—that instead of an immoral, sinful relationship as her church had taught, it was a healthy and loving relationship. She began counseling with a minister and sought legal counsel to protect her rights.

By this time, Sharon could respond to simple questions with finger movements or by squeezing Karen's hand, and later by typing. She was asked repeatedly to name the person she wanted to live with and have responsibility for her care and the answer was always the same: Karen. Karen's lawyer helped her to file for guardianship of Sharon in March 1984. Donald Kowalski immediately counterfiled, requesting that he be named sole guardian of Sharon. These events led to years of court hearings and the guardianship battle became quite public. Karen had to deal with coming out to her family, with learning about lesbian and gay legal issues, with public appearances on national TV, and with mounting legal fees. The courts were not kind to her. In October 1984, the Kowalskis filed a restraining order against Karen and restricted her visits. In July 1985, they were able to completely deny visitation and moved Sharon to a nursing home without good rehabilitation facilities.

Throughout the court proceedings, judges consistently ignored Sharon's wishes, even though several psychologists found her to be competent to make decisions for herself—she was considered totally helpless and the wishes of her father were always chosen over her own. No one recognized the validity of Karen and Sharon's relationship, although several health care providers acknowledged that Sharon responded best to Karen and was recovering at a faster pace than anticipated under Karen's guidance. Sharon's short-term memory was quite poor, and she did not remember why Karen was not visiting anymore—she became extremely depressed and began to regress in physical skills without Karen's emotional and physical care. Her family was embarrassed by her physical disability, never took her out of the nursing home on passes, and visited only rarely.

From August 1985 to January 1989, Karen continued her battle to see Sharon, and was finally allowed to visit Sharon after more than three years of separation. Subsequently, Karen was named as her guardian, when Sharon's family admitted that they could not provide optimal care. But the years of separation had taken their toll and Sharon remains severely disabled. This story is tragic from many angles—disability rights advocates were appalled by the lack of attention to Sharon's mental competence and stated wishes for her own care, by the consistent rulings by judges that Sharon not be allowed to testify in court proceedings, and by the privileging of her father's wishes over her own. Lesbian, gay, and bisexual rights advocates were appalled by the lack of acknowledgment of same-sex relationships. No legal spouse would have had to wage this kind of legal battle with parents, nor would she/he have been denied visitation rights. Finally, from a health care perspective, considerable potential for recovery was lost when Sharon was inappropriately moved to an inadequate facility without the emotional and physical support of her significant other. This is a book that should be read by all health care providers (see Thompson & Andrzejewski, 1988). Many of the issues raised by this story will also be addressed here, including the fears and concerns of partners of critically ill lesbian, gay, or bisexual people and the potentially harmful institutional practices and individual prejudices that impact on their health care.

How Many Lesbian, Gay, and Bisexual People Are There?

Because Americans are somewhat obsessed with labeling and counting things and people, much attention has been directed to statistical and other numerical surveys. Census surveys include questions about race, gender, and age, but ascertaining sexual or cultural identity is another issue entirely. Race is likely to be a visible, physical difference that is easy to identify (although this is not always true). Sexual identity, however, is invisible, and unless a person states that she/he is lesbian, gay, or bisexual, there is no way of knowing for sure. Since people can lose jobs, families, housing, or even their lives by disclosing their sexual identity, few are likely to reveal this information in a face-to-face interview, a telephone interview, or even a seemingly anonymous mail-in survey.

Another problem lies in the terminology and how and what you ask about sexuality. There are three basic methods of ascertaining sexual attractions: self-report, actual behavior, and measurement of physiological arousal. The latter method involves attaching some apparatus to a person's genitals and measuring penile tumesence or vaginal lubrication in response to pictures of people of the other sex, same sex, or both (Gonsiorek & Weinrich, 1991). In addition to being impractical, physiological arousal is rarely used because it might identify people who have fantasized about sex with a same-sex partner but have never actually acted on it, or never intend to act on their fantasies. Thus, this method would tend to overestimate the number of people with same-sex orientations. The other two methods, ascertaining self-identity or actual behavior are widely used, but not identical. If you ask whether respondents consider themselves lesbian, gay, bisexual, or heterosexual, you might obtain a different answer than if you ask, "Have you ever had sex with someone of the same sex as you?" For example, some people who have frequent same-sex sexual encounters label themselves as heterosexual (Kinsey, Pomeroy, & Martin, 1948). The first hint of this difference between behavior and identity and of the broad continuum of sexual experience was found in Alfred Kinsey's research in the 1940s and 1950s (Kinsey, Pomeroy, & Martin, 1948; Kinsey, Pomeroy, Martin, & Gebhard, 1953). The often repeated statement that approximately 10% of the total population are homosexual derives from the Kinsey data. Figure 1.1 shows Kinsey's 0 to 6 scale of sexual experience. Using the most conservative figures, Kinsey reported that about 90% of the population was entirely heterosexual, and that the remaining 10% had some degree of homosexual experience. Of course, Kinsey's data have been widely criticized because he based his ratings on people's actual behavior rather than on what they call themselves. People who have had one homosexual experience in adolescence are certainly not the same as people who have had exclusively same-sex experiences and relationships for their entire lives. On the other hand, homosexuality was even more hidden and stigmatized during the 1940s and 1950s than it is today, so the fact that so many people

Legend: 0 = entirely heterosexual
         1 = largely heterosexual, but with incidental homosexual history
         2 = largely heterosexual, but with distinct homosexual history
         3 = equally heterosexual and homosexual
         4 = largely homosexual, but with distinct heterosexual history
         5 = largely homosexual, but with incidental heterosexual history
         6 = entirely homosexual

Kinsey Scale Points

Sex	0	1	2	3	4	5	6
Women (%)	61–90	11–20	6–14	4–11	3–8	2–6	1–3
Men (%)	53–92	18–42	13–38	9–32	7–26	5–22	3–16

FIGURE 1.1.   Kinsey's continuum of sexual behavior. These figures vary depending on the age, educational level, race, and marital status of the respondents.

claimed same-sex sexual experiences was quite remarkable. For this reason, some people also think Kinsey's data underestimate the actual number of lesbian, gay, and bisexual people.

Studies since Kinsey have generally reported a somewhat smaller number, partly because most of them rely on self-reported identity than actual behavior, or they use more stringent criteria for rating a person's behavior. For example, Gebhard (1972) suggested that the frequency of exclusive homosexuality was 2%–5% (he did not count bisexuals or people with some heterosexual experience, which leaves out many people who self-identify as lesbian, gay, or bisexual but may have had considerable heterosexual experience in the past). Hatfield (1989), from data obtained by telephone interview, found that 6% of national respondents and 10% of respondents in San Francisco identified themselves as lesbian, gay, or bisexual. A large, cross-cultural study of men in France, the United Kingdom, and the United States (Sell et al., 1990) found that 5%–11% of respondents reported recent same-sex sexual behavior, and over their lifetimes, 8%–12% had same-sex experiences. Notably, the studies reviewed here are recognized for their methodological soundness and use of techniques with demonstrated "scientific" reliability and validity. In general, the studies that base their estimates on actual sexual behavior of people tend to report higher numbers than studies that ask people if they consider themselves lesbian, gay, bisexual, or heterosexual.

Other studies, less scientific and more politically motivated, also exist. Paul Cameron and his associates (e.g., Cameron, 1988; Cameron, Proctor, Coburn, & Forde, 1985), for example, have published this sort of work (see Gonsiorek & Weinrich, 1991). Expelled from the American Psychological Association for conducting unethical research on homosexuality, Cameron continues to publish in some medical journals today such as Lancet and the Nebraska Medical Journal. Cameron's goal is to underestimate the numbers of lesbian, gay, and bisexual people in order to make them appear as an insignificant minority, or to inflate the figures of HIV/AIDS among gay and bisexual men. For example, if 50% of the AIDS cases in the United States are gay or bisexual men, but only 2%–4% of the population is gay or bisexual, that presents a very different picture than if 10%–15% of the population is gay or bisexual. However, Cameron's finding that 2% of the population is gay, and 2% is bisexual, is so methodologically flawed as to make his figures useless, except perhaps for those with agendas motivated by other than scientific interest. However, the lay press does not recognize when research is poorly done and Cameron's work often makes headlines.

Gonsiorek and Weinrich (1991) reviewed studies of prevalence and concluded that the rate of homosexuality in the United States is somewhere between the 4%–17% mark, depending on whether bisexuals are included and how homosexuality is defined. But the actual number is not really that important. Whether 1 in 10 or 1 in 20 clients/patients is lesbian, gay, or bisexual, the health care provider needs to understand issues of sexual identity.

ORGANIZATION OF THIS BOOK

In Chapter 2 of this book I will provide factual information about lesbian, gay, and bisexual people in the United States and will introduce issues that are relevant to health care providers. These issues include discussion of concepts such as homophobia, internalized homophobia, heterosexism, "coming out" (adopting a label or identifying oneself as lesbian, gay, or bisexual), diversity within lesbian, gay, and bisexual communities and families, and speculations about the origins of sexual identity. Chapter 3 addresses common stereotypes about lesbian, gay, and bisexual people, with examples of the harm these stereotypes can inflict. Factual information based on recent empirical research will be provided to counter the stereotypes. Research about lesbian, gay, and bisexual relationships and families will be reviewed in Chapter 4. In the aftermath of the early 1990s, when "family values" was the buzzword for political campaigns, I will explore how same-sex couples forge family relationships. Lesbian, gay, and bisexual people have always been part of families—they have families of origin and they also create families from their significant others and friends. Often these families include children.

Chapter 5 will address attitudes of health care providers and explore how negative attitudes might impact health care delivery. I will explore some methods for reducing negative attitudes among health care providers. In Chapter 5, I will also examine some of the research on disclosure of sexual identity to a health care provider, and discuss some of the potential negative ramifications of disclosure. Chapter 6 addresses common developmental transitions of lesbian, gay, and bisexual people across the lifespan. In Chapters 7 and 8, I will explore potential health problems of lesbian and bisexual women and gay and bisexual men, respectively. In an ideal society, there would be few health risk differences between heterosexual women and men, and lesbian, gay, and bisexual people. However, experiences of harassment, discrimination, and other forms of oppression can create unique health problems that health care providers need to learn to recognize and treat. In Chapter 9, I will explore ways to avoid the tragedy that Karen Thompson experienced in her struggle to remain a part of her lover's life. This chapter emphasizes the creation of a nonoppressive health care practice. This practice includes use of inclusive language and hospital policies, creating a safe environment for lesbian, gay, and bisexual clients/patients and their families, and learning to be an advocate for lesbian, gay, and bisexual health care rights.

Each chapter will conclude with some type of exercise designed to expand your thinking about sexual identity, assess your own beliefs and attitudes, or apply the new knowledge to your own life.

EXERCISE: DETERMINING YOUR OWN SEXUAL IDENTITY

Klein, Sepekoff, and Wolf (1985) developed a scale to measure the multiple aspects of sexual identity. They suggested that sexual identity is broader than just sexual behavior, and proposed seven dimensions of human relationships that constitute sexual identity. This scale considers what sex (male or female) you prefer for each of the seven dimensions, and also, the sexual identity (mostly heterosexual, mostly lesbian or gay, or bisexual) you prefer in a partner. To measure your own sexual identity, look at the following two grids—fill in the first one based on the sex of the person you prefer for each of the seven dimensions, and the second grid based on the sexual identity of the person you prefer for each activity. For each dimension, rate your past, present, and ideal behavior.

Now examine the patterns displayed in each grid. Compare your past behavior to your present and your present behavior to your ideal. Do they match? If not, what can you do to make them match? How can you achieve your ideal sexual identity? Are you regularly exposed to people with different sexual identities than yourself? This scale works well because it does not define bisexuality, homosexuality or

Grid 1. The sex you prefer. Put a number from 1 to 7 in each space of the grid.

1	2	3	4	5	6	7
other sex only	other sex mostly	other sex somewhat more	both sexes equally	same sex somewhat more	same sex mostly	same sex only

Dimension	Past	Present	Ideal
Sexual Attraction			
Sexual Behavior			
Sexual Fantasies			
Emotional Preference			
Social Preference			
Self-Identification or Self-Image			
Lifestyle (person with whom you like to spend most of your time)			

Grid 2. The sexual identities of people you prefer for each dimension.

1	2	3	4	5	6	7
hetero only	hetero mostly	hetero somewhat more	hetero and gay equally	gay somewhat more	gay mostly	gay only

Dimension	Past	Present	Ideal
Sexual Attraction			
Sexual Behavior			
Sexual Fantasies			
Emotional Preference			
Social Preference			
Self-Identification or Self-Image			
Lifestyle (person with whom you like to spend most of your time)			

heterosexuality as matters only of sex, but as identities that encompass social and emotional dimensions as well. We have long recognized this fact of heterosexuality, but lesbian, gay, and bisexual identities are often thought of as exclusively matters of sex. This grid also demonstrates that there is often no clear line between lesbian, gay, bisexual, and heterosexual.

CHAPTER TWO

Lesbian, Gay, and Bisexual Issues

*IT WAS WITH EXTREME PRECAUTION that I came to know myself. I
had concluded, as a young boy, that there was a part of me that
I did not want to be; but there was nothing I could do. Almost
all of my life I felt like a drone, following some set path toward
my future, not living, but operating according to some prepro-
grammed specifications . . . . The day I graduated from high
school, I made a pact with myself to "come out" on campus before returning home for winter break. I had no fears. I had
come this far and didn't care what anyone else might think of
me. My parents knew I was gay, which I considered a plus, but
being typical black parents, they first berated me, then alienated me, then sent me to a psychologist to be cured. The local
Baptist minister was called in to scare the sickness out of me. (If
there had been any sickness there, believe me, he would have
scared it out.) My parents have simmered down since then, but
I am not sure they accept my sexuality; we simply don't discuss
it. (Calvin Glenn, 1991, pp. 47–48)*

In this chapter, I will present a range of factual information on lesbian, gay, and bisexual people and issues. After a brief historical
overview, demonstrating the recency of the concept of homosexuality
and exploring the progress that has been made in the past 25 years, I
will review some basic concepts toward a foundation for understanding lesbian, gay, and bisexual health care issues. Understanding of
these concepts, such as homophobia, heterosexism, coming out, and
diversity within lesbian, gay, and bisexual communities, is crucial for

17

anyone who works with sexual minorities because they have direct implications for physical and mental health. Finally, a discussion of the origins of sexual identity will conclude the chapter.

HISTORICAL OVERVIEW

Although descriptions of same-sex sexual behaviors can be found throughout recorded history, the concept of the lesbian, gay, or bisexual as a particular kind of person is a modern invention (D'Emilio & Freedman, 1988; Foucault, 1969). Prior to the early 1900s, same-sex *behaviors* were recognized and often punished, but there was no concept of a homosexual *person;* that is, sexual behaviors did not define a particular kind of person, but were thought to be potentials of any person. The word *homosexual* first appeared in the medical literature in 1869, and referred to a form of mental illness or deviant sexuality (an abnormal and excessive interest in people of the same sex). The term *heterosexual* appeared in the United States in a medical journal in 1892, and also originally referred to a mental illness—an abnormal and excessive interest in people of the other sex (Katz, 1995). Early sexologists, such as Sigmund Freud, Albert Ellis, and Richard von Krafft-Ebing published numerous case histories and theories speculating upon the origins of homosexuality, but rarely upon the origins of heterosexuality (Freud is the exception here). Thus, they advanced the idea that homosexuality needed explanation, but that heterosexuality did not; that heterosexuality was the norm and that homosexuality constituted the abnormal.

Most early research on homosexuality focused on adults who were being treated for mental illnesses, who sought therapy to cure them of their same-sex desires, or who were in prisons or mental institutions (Gonsiorek, 1991). Not surprisingly, this research found the homosexual to be poorly adjusted, immature, desperate, and secretive (e.g., Bergler, 1956; Socarides, 1975; Turner, Pielmaier, James, & Orwin, 1974). One psychoanalyst reacted violently against Kinsey's assertions in the 1940s and 1950s that homosexuality was a natural and relatively common form of sexual expression. Bergler asserted, "Homosexuality is not the 'way of life' these sick people gratuitously assume it to be, but a neurotic distortion of the total personality" (1956, p. 9). Bergler was even more negative about bisexuality when he claimed:

bisexuality—a state that has no existence beyond the word it-self—is an out-and-out fraud. . . . The theory claims that a man can be—alternately or concomitantly—homo and heterosexual. The statement is as rational as one declaring that a man can at the same time have cancer and perfect health. (p. 89)

In the scientific community, more objective, empirically based scientists began to side with Kinsey while the more psychoanalytic psychiatrists resented the intrusion into "their" domain, and continued to propose that homosexuality resulted from deviant childhood development. Although psychoanalysts in the United States were mostly negative about homosexuality, this idea did not stem directly from Freud. In 1935, Freud responded to a woman who wrote to him asking for help with her son. Freud wrote:

Homosexuality is assuredly no advantage but it is nothing to be ashamed of, no vice, no degradation, it cannot be classified as an illness; we consider it to be a variation of the sexual function produced by a certain arrest of sexual development. Many highly respectable individuals of ancient and modern times have been homosexuals, several of the greatest men among them (Plato, Michelangelo, Leonardo da Vinci, etc.). It is a great injustice to persecute homosexuality as a crime and a cruelty too. . . . By asking me if I can help, you mean, I suppose, if I can abolish homosexuality and make normal heterosexuality take its place. The answer is, in a general way, we cannot promise to achieve it. (Freud, 1935, in Katz, 1983, p. 506)

While debates about homosexuality raged in the medical community, other changes were occurring in society.

Following World War II, with the increase in population of urban areas, especially port cities, homosexual "communities" began to emerge, though they often consisted primarily of bars, "cruising areas," and small secretive social networks. Gay bars were routinely raided by police and extorted by organized crime. Homosexuals could not be open about their relationships and many lived in fear of discovery. For example, in the late 1950s in Chicago, a 17-year-old homosexual teenager, Craig, was walking to the subway with a 30-year-old man with whom he had just had consensual sex. Suddenly they were surrounded by four police cars—the police separated Craig and Frank, his older companion, and Frank had to stand trial. The prosecutor attempted to prove that Frank gave Craig money in exchange for sex, but Craig adamantly denied it. Despite Craig's denial and the lack of any evidence, Frank was sent to jail for five years on a charge of a "crime against nature." Craig was threatened with reform school, but due to his mother's pleading received a sentence of two years' probation with the condition that he see a psychiatrist. A few years later, Craig was arrested again, this time on a gay beach because he failed to wear a towel over his bathing suit. He was severely beaten by the police and spent three days in jail (Duberman, 1993).

In 1957, Evelyn Hooker's landmark study on identifying homosexuality by psychological test was published. A well-respected psychologist of the day, Hooker gave a series of psychological tests to 60 employed men who had not been diagnosed with any form of mental illness: half were gay and half were heterosexual. She then asked leading experts on these tests whether they thought the tests would enable them to distinguish homosexuals from heterosexuals, to which they answered, "Yes." However, when given the actual test results, the experts did no better than chance at identifying the homosexual men. Hooker concluded that, since no major psychological test could distinguish the gay men from heterosexual men, homosexuality per se could not be a mental illness. In fact, she suggested that societal stigmatization was the problem, not homosexuality. Hooker's findings were subsequently confirmed by dozens of studies that followed in the 1960s and later. Homosexuals could not be distinguished from heterosexuals on the basis of the following measures:

- General psychological characteristics (LaTorre & Wendenburg, 1983; McDaniel, 1989; Nurius, 1983).
- Self-concept or self-esteem (Carlson & Baxter, 1984; Carlson & Steuer, 1985; Christie & Young, 1986; Clark, 1975; Harry, 1983).
- Rates of psychiatric problems (Pillard, 1988; Saghir & Robins, 1973; Saghir, Robins, Walbran, & Gentry, 1970a, 1970b; Weinberg & Williams, 1974).

The only consistent differences between homosexuals and heterosexuals have been in rates of depression and suicide attempts, particularly in the adolescent years (Bell & Weinberg, 1978; Gibson, 1994;

Kourany, 1987; Roesler & Deisher, 1972; Saunders & Valente, 1987); and in rates of alcohol abuse (Finnegan & McNally, 1987; Kus, 1995). I will discuss depression, suicide attempts, and substance abuse in more detail in a later chapter, as these complex issues may be related more to the degree of acceptance of a homosexual identity and to external stressors than to any underlying psychopathology. Some authors have found that although homosexuals as a group make more suicide attempts than heterosexuals, the rate of completed suicide is comparable to heterosexuals (Buhrich & Loke, 1988; Rich, Fowler, Young, & Blenkush, 1986).

As the research was changing and finding no adverse effects of homosexuality, massive societal changes were also occurring. The 1960s were an era marked by political/social change and liberation movements. Sparked by the civil rights movement and women's liberation organizations, "gay liberation" was born. Many people point to a single event in 1969 that served as a catalyst (e.g., Duberman, 1993). The Stonewall Inn, a working-class gay bar in Greenwich Village, had experienced more than its share of police harassment over the years, and usually police raids resulted in docile arrests. However, one night in June 1969, the patrons fought back and rioting broke out in the streets for several nights afterward. Within months, dozens of gay liberation groups formed all over the country. Modeled after black civil rights movements, gay liberation used rallies, sit-ins, demonstrations, and other visible forms of protest to make its issues known. This political organizing also brought people together socially, and communities with distinct subcultures began to emerge in many U.S. cities.

In 1973, under pressure from gay rights groups and from the growing psychological research that found homosexuals to be no different from heterosexuals on the majority of psychological measures, the American Psychiatric Association removed homosexuality from the *Diagnostic and Statistical Manual of Mental Disorders (DSM).* It did retain a diagnosis referred to as "Egodystonic Homosexuality," which was used for the person who was unhappy with her/his sexual identity and wished to change. MacDonald (1976) noted that before 1973, one was sick if she/he liked being homosexual, but after 1973, one was sick only if she/he did not like being homosexual. Eventually, even the egodystonic diagnosis proved too vague and the futility of attempting to change sexual identity even in motivated patients led to its removal from the *DSM* in 1986. The 1980s were an era of increased tolerance within the psychological community, leading to more therapies that helped lesbian, gay, and bisexual people cope with a difficult life rather than trying to cure them. However, some therapists continued to hold negative attitudes and "reparative" therapies can still be found today (see Chapter 3 for a critique of these therapy methods and Haldeman, 1994, for a review of the research). There are still some therapists (and health care professionals) who believe that the decision to remove homosexuality from the fourth edition of the *Diagnostic and Statistical Manual of Mental Disorders (DSM*-4, American Psychiatric Association, 1994) was a political one, prompted by pressure by gay rights organizations. However, a review of the scientific literature clearly supports the view that homosexuality does not constitute a mental illness.

Other signs of change during the 1970s and 1980s could be found in many different segments of society. Some states and local municipalities began to include sexual orientation in their human rights or nondiscrimination statements. Gay student groups appeared on nearly every major college campus in the country. Magazines, newspapers, and even television began to include stories about gay events or people, and a growing number of publications targeted gay audiences. Many gay people sought out safer, more anonymous living arrangements and settled in urban neighborhoods, creating "gay ghettos" in some of the larger U.S. cities. All these societal changes began to make it easier for some homosexuals to live more openly, thus becoming a more visible presence in U.S. society. At the same time, some changes in terminology began to occur. Some activists refused to accept a label tainted with abnormality (homosexual), and chose to use an old code word long used within the homosexual community to identify members (gay).

The gay liberation movements of the 1970s were profoundly influenced by the civil rights and women's movements. Many women who were active in both gay and women's groups were enraged by the sexism in the gay male community and discouraged by the homophobia of the women's community. They demanded changes in both groups, asserting that lesbian and bisexual issues were priorities for women's organizations and that women's issues were priorities for gay organizations. Many felt excluded from both groups, noting that "gay" meant men and "women" meant heterosexual. By the late 1970s, most gay organizations had adopted names like "gay and lesbian" to indicate their inclusiveness, and women's organizations began to include lesbian issues in their agendas. However, some lesbians remained disillusioned and formed separatist lesbian-feminist organizations.

A similar process occurred in the 1980s, when bisexuals came "out of the closet" and demanded inclusion in the organizations they had helped to create. Thus, many groups became "gay, lesbian, and bisexual." The trend in the 1990s is for organizations to become more inclusive of the needs of transgendered people (people who believe that their bodies and psychological gender do not match, or who feel that the idea of only two genders is too limiting and does not apply to them). In the dynamic history of "gay" political organizing, terminology is constantly changing and there are no universally accepted labels. Some people, both women and men, continue to call themselves "homosexuals." Some women prefer gay to lesbian, some prefer "queer," and others refuse labels altogether. However, the most widely used terminology used to refer to individuals is "gay, lesbian, or bisexual." When referring to the phenomena of same-sex relationships or orientations in a collective way, "homosexuality" is still widely used.

The invention of the "modern homosexual" by psychiatrists of the late nineteenth century has had both positive and negative effects. The increased attention given to people with same-sex desires created a forum for them to learn about others with similar feelings, and allowed them to establish an identity based on that similarity. Until someone named homosexuality and put it into the popular discourse, it could not form the basis for a community or a political identity. When there is a label for a person's feelings or desires, she/he feels validated and less alienated; the person then knows that there are others with similar feelings.

On the other hand, the harm inflicted by the medical profession in labeling homosexuality as a mental illness and developing (and using) a variety of treatments to "cure" homosexuality has had devastating effects (Silverstein, 1991). According to Katz (1992):

Among the treatments are surgical measures: castration, hysterectomy, and vasectomy. In the 1800s, surgical removal of the ovaries and of the clitoris are discussed as a "cure" for various forms of female "erotomania," including, it seems, Lesbianism. Lobotomy was performed as late as 1951. A variety of drug therapies have been employed, including the administration of

*hormones, LSD, sexual stimulants, and sexual depressants. Hyp-
nosis, used on Gay people in America as early as 1899, was still
being used to treat such "deviant behavior" in 1967. Other
documented "cures" are shock treatment, both electrical and
chemical; aversion therapy, employing nausea-inducing drugs,
electric shock, and/or negative verbal suggestion; and a type of
behavior therapy called "sensitization," intended to increased
heterosexual arousal, making ingenuous use of pornographic
photos. Often homosexuals have been the subject of Freudian
psychoanalysis and other varieties of individual and group psychotherapy. (p. 129)*

Many gay, lesbian, and bisexual people were forcibly incarcerated in
mental institutions and treated without their consent, and some of the
therapies, as in the following case, were particularly dangerous to
their physical and/or mental health:

*Aversion therapy was conducted with a male homosexual who
had a heart condition. The particular form of aversion therapy
involved creation of nausea, by means of an emetic accompanied by talking about his homosexuality. . . . In this case, the patient died as a result of a heart attack brought on by the use of
the emetic. (Weinberg & Bell, 1972, p. 287)*

Although these experiences of forced treatment or incarceration
occur less frequently to adults today, lesbian, gay, and bisexual teens
are still vulnerable to commitment by their parents. These negative experiences, coupled with the misuse of research to promote or perpetuate discrimination, led to a generalized distrust of medicine and health
care institutions in general in many lesbian, gay, and bisexual people.
The legacy left by early psychiatrists, and maintained by prejudiced
health care providers today, constitutes a major barrier to quality
health care in the 1990s.

Basic Terminology

Before proceeding, I need to define some terms that I will use
throughout the book. First, although we use the terms sex and gender
almost interchangeably in our culture, they have slightly different

meanings. In this book, *sex* will be defined as the biological markers that distinguish females and males, such as external genitalia, chromosomes, and internal reproductive organs. Usually, sex determination is based only on external genitalia—few of us have chromosome tests or X-rays of our internal organs to determine our sex. *Gender* refers to the socially constructed views of femininity and masculinity—what you should wear, act like, and think like if you are female or male in our culture. In U.S. culture, sex is supposed to determine both people's gender and their attraction to members of the other sex (I don't use the term *opposite sex,* because women's and men's bodies are much more alike than different, so "opposite" doesn't really describe the differences well and it sets up the idea that there are two different species of humans who are opposites in more ways than just parts of their genitalia).

You might have noticed that the media use at least two different terms to refer to the sexuality of a person: sexual orientation and sexual preference. A sexual *orientation* is considered to be determined from birth or at a very early age, then remains stable throughout the rest of life. An orientation is generally considered to be biological in nature; that is, people are born heterosexual, lesbian, gay, or bisexual, or have a deeply ingrained psychological sense of their sexuality from a very early age (Gonsiorek & Weinrich, 1991). A sexual *preference* implies some degree of choice or flexibility. Preferences are not biological and can be changed fairly easily. Gay rights activists are likely to use sexual orientation when arguing for basic human rights, and to argue that there is no evidence that people can change their sexuality easily (the psychological literature clearly shows that this is true). Those who oppose gay rights are more likely to use sexual preference, and promote the idea that people who want to change their sexuality can do so via religion or strong moral character. Since we don't really know whether sexuality is inborn and biological or is influenced more strongly by environmental factors and personal choice (more on this later), I will use a more neutral term in this book. Sexual *identity* is the way that an individual labels and interprets her/his own sexual attractions and behaviors. At this point in time, we have four fairly well-recognized sexual identities: heterosexual, lesbian, gay, and bisexual. Some people argue that asexual should also be included, acknowledging that some people have no sexual attractions. A person can be celibate (choose not to be sexually active) and still have a sexual identity, demonstrating that asexual and celibate are not the same thing.

This discussion of sexual identities becomes more complicated if you consider the basis for the definitions. Do we base our definitions on the identities people claim for themselves (what they call themselves), on their actual behavior (what they do), or on their physiological arousal patterns, dreams, or fantasies (what turns them on)? Each one of these might differ in the same person. Can a man be gay if he has never had sex with a man? Is a woman still heterosexual if she is happily married to a man, but has occasional fantasies about making love to a woman? Our definitions of sexuality are far from clear-cut and demonstrate the fluidity of sexuality in people's lives. Most studies use the self-identity definition—lesbians, gay men, and bisexuals are people who use one of those labels to describe themselves.

Some people confuse the terms *sexual identity* and *gender identity.* Gender identity refers to the sense of self as male or female, masculine or feminine. There are some people who feel that their physical bodies do not match their psychological gender; for example, a biological woman may feel that she is psychologically male. People with this mismatch between biological and psychological gender are called transsexuals, or transgendered people. Some decide to have medical and surgical treatments that make their bodies more closely match their psychological identity, but the majority do not have "sex change" operations. Transgendered people can be heterosexual, lesbian, gay, or bisexual in their sexual identities. The majority of lesbian, gay, and bisexual people have bodies and psychological genders that match, and they are not interested in changing their biological sex. However, some lesbian, gay, and bisexual people are interested in broadening our ideas about gender and allowing all people to express themselves freely regardless of gender. Many lesbian, gay, and bisexual people are "gender benders."

Lifestyle is another term often applied to lesbian, gay, and bisexual people. But just what is a "bisexual lifestyle?" This term is inappropriate when referring to an individual's sexual identity. A lifestyle is a pattern of exercising, dietary habits, health practices, and stress management, as in "healthy lifestyle," and is not unique to sexual identity. Some lesbian, gay, and bisexual people have healthy lifestyles and some do not, just like heterosexual people. To suggest that there is a unique lesbian, gay, or bisexual lifestyle is to deny the diversity of patterns of living and coping within these groups.

Homophobia

Since the objective scientific studies from the 1960s on have confirmed that lesbian, gay, and bisexual people cannot be distinguished from heterosexuals on nearly any measure of personality or emotional adjustment, why are lesbian, gay, and bisexual people feared, hated, and avoided? In 1972, psychologist George Weinberg introduced the term *homophobia* into the scientific literature. This term, defined as an irrational fear of homosexuals, put the onus for negative attitudes where it belonged—on the people with the negative attitudes rather than on its victims. However, the term has its share of problems. First, in psychological terms, a phobia is an irrational fear that results in a physiological fight-or-flight syndrome (sweaty palms, racing heart, dilated pupils, increased blood pressure, feelings of anxiety). Attitudes about lesbian, gay, or bisexual people rarely fit that precise definition (Haaga, 1991). Specifically, hatred (Card, 1990), discomfort, disapproval (Eliason & Raheim, 1996), anger, or guilt (Ernulf & Innala, 1987) are more often the motivating factors than fear. With a true phobia, people are motivated to change because the phobia is uncomfortable and they recognize that the fears are irrational. Homophobic people are rarely motivated to change; they generally do not believe that their attitudes are irrational (Card, 1990). Despite these flaws, however, the term homophobia has gained widespread usage.

Current attempts to describe negative attitudes about lesbian, gay, and bisexual people indicate that attitudes exist on a continuum from very positive to very negative, and may include a set of reactions that are qualitatively different (Ernulf & Innala, 1987). Eliason (1996a) and Eliason and Raheim (1996) found a wide variety of attitudes that may stem from different underlying factors. These attitudes are described in the following list, along with some actual examples of comments made by heterosexual respondents on a survey of the campus climate for lesbian, gay, and bisexual people at a major midwestern university (Eliason, 1993a):

1. *Celebration.* This attitude proposes that lesbian, gay, and bisexual people are unique and should be cherished, or at the very least, recognized for the contributions they make to society. Examples of celebration comments included:
   - Gay people are part of the social fabric of America—they need to be portrayed as healthy folks with a different orientation

who do not represent a hateful threat to American values, but simply a broadening of them.

- It is so tragic to see people having difficulty accepting other people who have consciously chosen to practice their innovative lifestyle, which they believe is the most rightful way of healthy living . . . I hope lesbian, gay, and bisexual rights will be recognized and cherished . . . soon.

2. *Acceptance.* People who fit into this category recognize that all people deserve equal rights regardless of any human characteristic such as race, gender, or sexual identity:

- I feel lesbian, gay, and bisexual people should be treated no differently than heterosexuals.
- There's no question American society has asinine attitudes about lesbian, gay, and bisexual people and racial minorities as well. It drags us all down and prohibits us from achieving greater heights as a people.

Some authors argue that acceptance is not really a positive category at all—why should sexual identity be something we need to accept? There is still an implication that lesbian, gay, and bisexual people have some significant difference from heterosexuals that requires their acceptance. Shouldn't all human beings be valued just on the basis of their humanity?

3. *Tolerance.* The first of the clearly negative categories, people who are tolerant are uncomfortable with lesbian, gay, and bisexual issues, but believe that people have a right to lead their lives as they choose—as long as they keep it private:

- No one should flaunt sexuality, regardless of preference.
- Sexual orientation should be a private matter and not shoved down one's throat.
- I don't think they [lesbian, gay, bisexual people] should be ashamed . . . but I don't go around town telling people I'm heterosexual.
- I have nothing against gays, but . . . I don't wear my sexuality on my sleeve and I don't bring my relationships into the workplace.

What people in this category don't realize is that heterosexuality is "shoved down our throats" every day. People do "flaunt" their heterosexuality by wearing engagement and wedding rings, putting their wedding and anniversary pictures in the newspaper, holding hands in public, posting a picture of a wife or husband on their desk, or even talking about what they did on the weekend with their spouses or dates. Lesbian, gay, and bisexual people are not asking for the right to have sex in public places, but rather, to be able to be open and honest about their relationships in the same ways that heterosexual people can express their relationships.

4. *Disapproval.* Some people disapprove of lesbian, gay, and bisexual relationships on the basis of religious beliefs:

   • God says I must love my brother and I do but God also says this lifestyle is wrong and I cannot condone it anyway. It is sin.
   • I clearly believe homosexuality is a sin and God punishes sin.
   • I believe God created the family to be headed by a male and female, anything other is abnormal.

I discuss religious beliefs and the Bible to condemn homosexuality in some detail in Chapter 3. Other people disapprove of homosexuality on the basis of the "unnaturalness" of same-sex relationships:

• I don't care who people have sex with, but it's unnatural to be other than heterosexual.
• I think anything other than heterosexualism is wrong. I believe it is a mental or emotional disorder and wonder if this is being studied. I wonder if it's treatable with therapy or medications or ECT [electroconvulsive therapy].

5. *Disgust.* The reaction of a small number of people comes close to fitting the psychological definition of a phobia. This group does not want any exposure to gay people or issues and has a negative emotional response to gay people:

   • I think what bothers most people is the actual sex act that occurs. It's totally gross to think about.
   • I find such lifestyles to be personally repugnant.
   • It is unnatural and appalling to me.

6. *Hatred.* A small, but extremely dangerous group of individuals despises gay people or feels threatened by homosexuality. Some of the people in this group are capable of violence:

- It is an insult to God himself. His view of same-sex partners is that it is an abomination. His reaction to it is utter destruction.
- Having been approached by queers in the past . . . I defended myself and ended up in jail. The first time . . . I was able to pound the crap out of the guy . . . the third time I knocked the person out.
- I hit one guy in the throat and broke another's car window for grabbing me.

People in the hatred category have been the most widely studied, since they commit the majority of hate crimes against lesbian, gay, and bisexual people. Research reveals that most are late adolescent and young adult men who go out in gangs looking for victims—many wait in parking lots of gay bars. They may use religion to justify their attacks although they are not otherwise religious (Comstock, 1991; Herek & Birrell, 1992).

Other elements of homophobia might include concern that rights given to lesbian, gay, or bisexual people will mean rights or benefits removed from some other group, such as heterosexuals or other minority groups. Similarly, some people believe that other groups are more deserving of rights and attention to their plight. Examples of this form of homophobia include:

- The attention directed to gays is blown out of proportion to the number on campus. It's like with handicapped persons—it's important to give them access, but the cost is way out of proportion.
- I feel middle-class people of no particular disadvantaged group are highly discriminated against, especially white middle-class males.
- Minority rights have always been at the expense of the majority . . . any minority group does not have to be really qualified to obtain any position . . . and they drain funds away from majority needs.
- I also feel heterosexuals can be discriminated against . . . examples include someone who frequents prostitutes, is into bondage, politicians who sleep around.

Viewing homophobia as a continuum that reflects a range of attitudes is important because special strategies may be needed for different kinds of attitudes. Whereas providing accurate information to dispel stereotypes may improve the attitude of the tolerant or even disapproving person, education alone is unlikely to change the attitude of the person who feels hatred. Those who disapprove on the grounds of religious beliefs may benefit from the research of recent Bible scholars, whereas those who disapprove based on the reproductive imperative (the idea that any sex which does not lead to procreation is unnatural) may benefit from discussions of the severing of the link between sex and reproduction in modern society. People who feel hatred may need empathy training to help them learn what the victim of a hate crime might experience.

Now take a minute to consider which of the preceding categories best describes your own beliefs. Think about your attitudes in the past, now, and ideally. If your beliefs have changed, think about why that has occurred. If you would like to change your attitudes further, how could you accomplish that goal?

What I have described in some detail is "personal homophobia," the negative beliefs and attitudes of individuals. Blumenfeld (1992) also discusses three other forms of homophobia that extend out from the individual:

1. *Interpersonal homophobia* occurs when individuals express their attitudes to other people, and can include ignoring, social rejection, name-calling, antigay jokes, verbal threats and intimidation, and physical violence.

2. *Institutional homophobia* refers to the systematic discrimination against lesbian, gay, or bisexual people by the government, educational systems, legal systems, and other major institutions of society. This is discussed further under the concept of heterosexism: It includes policies and laws that actively exclude lesbian, gay, and bisexual people, or render them invisible by assuming that all people are heterosexual.

3. *Cultural homophobia* includes the societal norms that legitimate discrimination. Cultural homophobia works through erasing lesbian, gay, and bisexual people from history books and in the current media, and allows even good, ethical people to stand aside and do nothing when antigay remarks or behaviors are made.

Blumenfeld also describes how homophobia hurts all people, not just lesbian, gay, and bisexual people:

- Homophobia locks people into rigid gender roles that deny creativity and individuality.
- Homophobic socialization in childhood and adolescence leads some heterosexuals to act in immoral and unethical ways, "dehumanizing" them.
- Homophobia prevents some people from forming strong emotional and intimate connections with people of the same sex for fear of being labeled as gay.
- Homophobia hurts families in many ways—some families reject gay members, other impose a silence on them, and many are embarrassed or ashamed to speak to friends about their gay family members. Some families feel guilty and wonder what they did wrong to cause homosexuality or bisexuality in a family member.
- Homophobia prevents schools from providing comprehensive sex education programs that would benefit all students. The opposition to teaching about sexual orientation in the public schools constrains all forms of sex education.
- Homophobia diverts energy from more productive activities. Lesbian, gay, and bisexual people expend much energy defending themselves from homophobia, and some heterosexuals spend inordinate time and energy engaged in hate crimes against lesbian, gay, and bisexual people.

Internalized Homophobia

Since we are socialized to some extent within the same homophobic culture, people who later in life identify as lesbian, gay, or bisexual also internalize those negative attitudes. A major function of the resocialization process called "coming out" (described later in this chapter), involves unlearning the negative stereotypes and learning the truth about oneself and other lesbian, gay, and bisexual people. The truth is that most lesbian, gay, and bisexual people are hardworking, good people who create healthy, loving, long-term relationships. But just like some heterosexuals, some lesbian, gay, and bisexual people come from dysfunctional homes, are boring, annoying, become violent in their relationships, or abuse substances. These are human tendencies or problems that are not directly linked to sexual identity.

During the resocialization process, internalized homophobia can have negative effects on a person's attitudes, behaviors, and relationships. Ariel Shidlo (1994) defined internalized homophobia as a "set of negative attitudes and affects toward homosexuality in other persons and toward homosexual features in oneself" (p. 178). The incorporation of this set of negative attitudes into a person's self-image disrupts normal development (Malyon, 1982). The consequences of internalized homophobia can include distrust, loneliness, under- and overachievement, impaired sexual functioning, difficulty forming intimate relationships, unsafe sexual experiences, alcohol and drug abuse, depression and suicide, and domestic violence. Like any kind of self-hatred, internalized homophobia can be turned inward to become self-destructive behaviors, or turned outward, in violence toward or pushing away of significant others.

The prevalence of internalized homophobia has not been carefully studied, but in one large-scale survey (over 1,000 lesbians and gay men), Bell and Weinberg (1978) found "guilt" about sexual experiences in 28% of the white gay men, 50% of black gay men, 20% of white lesbians, and 33% of black lesbians. About one-fourth of the sample considered homosexuality to be an emotional disorder (this study was conducted very early in the gay liberation movement). Attempts to measure conscious aspects of internalized homophobia, such as shame and guilt, might overlook unconscious defense mechanisms including rationalization, denial, projection, and distorted thinking about sexuality (Shidlo, 1994).

Heterosexism

The concept of homophobia focuses on individual attitudes or prejudices. Many theorists have pointed out the limitations of this approach (e.g., Kitzinger, 1987) because negative attitudes are also embedded into systems of society such as the media, religion, legal discourses, education, and health care. To address this systemic oppression, Morin (1977) proposed the term *heterosexism* (also called cultural homophobia). Heterosexism is the belief that heterosexuality is the only normal or natural option for human relationships and/or that heterosexuality is superior to homosexuality. Heterosexism is evident in everyday life.

TV programs promote heterosexuality by presenting only male-female relationships as having validity. If lesbian, gay, or (rarely) bisexual persons appear on a TV program or in a movie, they are often shown as mentally ill *(Silence of the Lambs)*, a psychopathic killer *(Basic Instinct)*, a neurotic or rather bizarre character (both the gay male and bisexual female characters on *Roseanne*), or as the source of the joke *(Married with Children, Coach, Murphy Brown, Frasier,* and dozens of other comedies that use lesbian, gay, or bisexual people for comic relief). Gay characters with serious, regular roles, such as the young man in *Melrose Place,* are not allowed the range of sexual expression that other characters have.

Another example of heterosexism is the marital status category that appears on many kinds of forms. Since a same-sex couple cannot be legally married in the United States (at least at the time of this writing—the Hawaii Supreme Court had still not ruled whether same-sex marriage would be allowed there), they cannot check the "married" box on a form, but to check "single," would be to deny their relationship. The marital status categories deny validity to cohabitating heterosexual couples as well. Marriage, a heterosexist institution, provides many special privileges such as tax breaks, child custody, and social validation to the elite who qualify.

Heterosexism is a parallel term to racism and sexism, and it operates in a similar manner. Figure 2.1 outlines this process. First, there are the dominant discourses of society that produce the knowledge of our culture: educational systems, religion, law, the media in all its forms, and health care. These discourses provide knowledge about lesbian, gay, and bisexual people that may be distorted, inaccurate, outdated, or even absent; for example, many high school sex education programs do not even mention that some people might be gay. Sedgwick (1990) described silence as a powerful form of knowledge: A topic that is taboo, or totally neglected, sends a strong message about its undesirability. Silence has been used to perpetuate prejudice about race, gender, and sexuality. A prime example is that until recent years, the history of people of African descent in the United States was conspicuously absent from most textbooks used in public schools, leading many to (incorrectly) assume that African Americans have made little or no contribution to U.S. history or culture. Likewise, many important historical figures who had significant same-sex relationships in their lives are portrayed in textbooks as heterosexual (e.g., King James of the

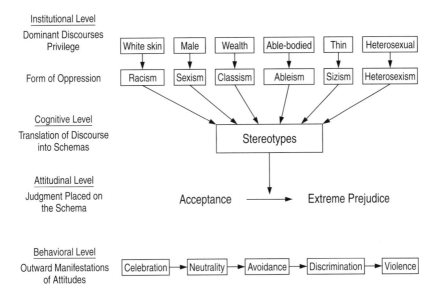

FIGURE 2.1. The relationship between dominant discourses of the United States and individual prejudices and behavior.

Bible translation fame, Michelangelo, Walt Whitman, Lawrence of Arabia, Eleanor Roosevelt, and many others).

The knowledge base that we learn as children, and rely on as adults, may consist of distorted stereotypes instead of accurate information. For example, discussion of lesbian, gay, or bisexual people in sex education programs might include some mention of child molestation, despite considerable evidence that perpetrators of childhood sexual abuse are heterosexual men more than 90% of the time (Jenny, Roesler, & Poyer, 1994). Discussions of heterosexuality may not include this link with child molestation, although it is sometimes appropriate to do so. Other sexual topics are taboo—not considered appropriate topics of discussion at all. For example, former Surgeon General Jocelyn Elders was dismissed from her post because she agreed that discussion of masturbation should be included in sex education programs in the schools. By not mentioning masturbation in sex education programs, we perpetuate the myth that masturbation is wrong or unnatural. Similarly, by not including discussions of homosexuality in sex education programs, we perpetuate the stereotype that homosexuality is unnatural, immoral, or limited to a few, deviant people.

Dominant discourses transmit stereotypes about groups of people that differ depending on the characteristics of the group (e.g., race, ethnicity, religion, gender, sexual identity, age), but stereotypes have some similar effects across these groups. For example, minority groups are often portrayed as less intelligent, less "human," and more primitive than the dominant group. Stereotypes about minorities often include a sexual component. For years, African American men have been stereotyped as rapists and African American women as promiscuous or as having greater sex drives than European American women. Asian men are cast as asexual or impotent, and Asian women as "china dolls" or submissive sex toys. Latinos are also stereotyped as more sensuous than European Americans, and stereotypes about the "primitive" sex practices of Native Americans were used to help justify annihilation of native people in the United States (D'Emilio & Freedman, 1988). Sexual stereotypes about lesbian, gay, and bisexual people include the idea that they are more promiscuous, more preoccupied with sex, engage in "deviant" sexual practices (often defined as nonprocreative), and are incapable of stable relationships. Lesbian, gay, and bisexual people who are also African American, Latino(a), Asian American, or Native American are subject to the combination of stereotypes by race and sexuality. That is, they experience racist stereotypes in both White heterosexual and gay, lesbian, and bisexual communities, and they experience homophobic attitudes in their racial communities.

Because the stereotypes from the dominant discourses circulate throughout the culture, children learn them at an early age, internalizing them into belief systems that take on affective undertones (emotions). For example, most people believe that child molestation is a despicable act. If you believe the stereotype that lesbian, gay, and bisexual people are child molesters, then they become despicable people. I will discuss common stereotypes about lesbian, gay, and bisexual people in detail in Chapter 3. When we apply some value judgment to a stereotype, we call it an attitude. Attitudes can range from very positive to very negative (as in the example provided earlier of the categories extending from celebration to hatred).

Behavior is the final component of this model: the ways by which we express our attitudes outwardly. Behaviors of prejudiced people can include avoidance of minority groups, feelings of discomfort when around members of minority groups, telling antiminority group jokes, making fun of minority group members, discriminating against minorities (denying jobs, housing, education, charging higher rent, etc.), harassment (verbal or physical threats, cross-burnings, swastikas, etc.), and violence (gay-bashing, hate crimes including destruction of private property, and murder). Heterosexism pervades our entire culture, making it extremely difficult for people to overcome their heterosexual (and heterosexist) socialization and choose a path that diverts from the norm. Yet a significant number of people do just that—they "come out" as lesbian, gay, or bisexual.

COMING OUT

An extensive literature has emerged in psychology about the coming out process—the circumstances by which a person decides to adopt a potentially stigmatizing label, such as lesbian, gay, or bisexual, and discloses that identity to at least one other person. Why would a person choose to risk loss of job, housing, and educational opportunities; rejection by family and friends; and potential harassment, physical harm, or even loss of life? The decision to identify as lesbian, gay, or bisexual is not a trivial one; it is the culmination of an agonizing, soul-searching process. As Del Martin and Phyllis Lyon (1972) noted:

> *I am a Lesbian. A simple statement, it would seem, which merely conveys that the woman expressing it has a preference for women both erotically and emotionally. But behind that statement may be years, sometimes decades of self doubt and guilt, and painful conflict—conflict between recognition of her inner being and acceptance of an assigned societal role, conflict between the desperate need for family support and despair at the prospect of bringing shame on her loved ones, conflict between her religious belief in God's eternal love for all His children and the negative pronouncements of church doctrine, conflict between celibacy and breaking the law, between honesty and deceit, between abject silence and open admission, between maintaining a dual life and loss of a career, between being crippled or whole, between life and death. (p. 21)*

Most of the following discussion applies primarily to lesbian and gay identity because it has been studied much more than bisexual identity. The literature includes two different kinds of models of coming out—linear or stage models (e.g., Cass, 1979; Chapman & Brannock, 1987; Minton & McDonald, 1984; Plummer, 1975) and nonlinear or cyclical models (Eliason, 1996b; Ponse, 1978; Troiden, 1988). Both approaches have merit, so a brief discussion of each kind will be presented. Understanding the stages of coming out is critical for health care providers because of the health implications, particularly during the early stages of this process.

Vivienne Cass (1979; 1984a, 1984b) proposed one of the earliest and best studied linear models of coming out. Based on her experiences as a therapist for lesbian and gay clients, she developed the following 6-stage model and then tested it empirically. The stages are as follows:

1. *Identity Confusion.* The person has certain experiences of sexual attractions that disrupt the self-identity as heterosexual, resulting in confusion. Some people deal with the confusion by totally rejecting the possibility of homosexuality, thus ending the process, whereas others may consider the option and begin to explore it.

2. *Identity Comparison.* The individual compares her/his own behavior and feelings with the societal notion of the homosexual. If the societal attitudes surrounding the person are too negative concerning homosexuality, the person may stop exploration at this point. Alternatively, she/he may decide to learn more by contacting a homosexual person or organization, or gathering more information.

3. *Identity Tolerance.* The person tries on the label "homosexual" for size, and has interactions with other homosexual persons. If these contacts are of good quality, the person can continue to grow. If they are bad experiences, exploration may stop. During this stage, many people lead separate lives and do not tell family or friends about their homosexual exploration.

4. *Identity Acceptance.* Positive experiences may lead to feelings of self-worth and self-acceptance. Selective disclosure of the homosexual identity often begins during this stage.

5. *Identity Pride.* In the face of negative attitudes and social stigmatization, but positive self-worth, the individual may reject some heterosexuals as too narrow-minded and become more

loyal and proud of homosexuals and her/his own homosexual identity.

6. *Identity Synthesis.* At this final point, the sexual identity becomes integrated into the total personality. Homosexuality becomes just one more aspect of the person, resulting in a sense of peace and inner harmony.

Cass (1984b) has tried to validate this model statistically, using survey data from 69 lesbians and 109 gay men. The results showed that many people did experience their coming out as a series of distinct stages, and that there were no differences between lesbians and gay men. However, the statistical approach looks at groups, not individuals, and it is likely that any given individual may have different experiences of coming out. In fact, Kahn (1991) assessed the model with data obtained from 81 lesbians, and reported that some skipped stages and others traversed the stages in different order. Kahn found five different patterns of progression through the stages. Sophie (1985/1986) also found different patterns of coming out in women, including a return to heterosexual identity for a few.

Another problem with Cass's model (as well as most of the other linear stage models) is that the sample did not include any bisexuals, thus did not provide data about bisexual identity development. In most of the early studies, bisexuals were lumped together with lesbians and gay men, or excluded from studies. Bisexuals are assumed to develop like lesbian and gay people, but there is little empirical data to warrant this assumption.

These linear stage models focus on the individual, interpsychic realm—how an individual in isolation comes to a sense of sexual identity. In reality, all of our identities are interrelated and social and historical factors greatly impact the coming out process. For example, knowledge that homosexuality exists may come from the media or the first feelings of difference may result from a sexual or highly emotional relationship with another person. Living in a period when lesbian, gay, and bisexual characters are appearing on TV on a more regular, if still compromised, basis may allow others to "discover" their difference at an earlier age than people who came out in the 1950s. Thus, the beginning point of the process may differ. Another problem with the linear models concerns context: No attention is given to other important human characteristics such as race, gender, age, and class background. Sexual identities do not form in isolation, but develop in relation to other human qualities and to other social beings.

Nevertheless, the stage models provide mental health clinicians and health care providers with some guidelines for the coming out process. Even though people may experience coming out in different ways, they may share some common feelings and experiences. Health care providers who are aware of these stages can have a better understanding of the person's perspective. For example, someone experiencing identity confusion—the first stage in this model—needs information rather than pressure to assume or commit to a sexual identity. A person in the later stages of identity tolerance may put her/himself at risk if experimenting with sexuality in an unprotected manner. Internalized homophobia may be common in most of the early stages of coming out.

Paula Rust (1992, 1993, 1996) has written about bisexual identity development, showing how it might differ from lesbian and gay experience, and highlighting the fluidity of sexuality. Initially, she critiques research that reduces the coming out process to discrete milestone events, such as reporting the average age at which respondents first felt different, or the average age at which they experienced their first same-sex attraction or sexual experience. According to Rust, using average ages obscures the wide variation in individuals and ignores the vast implications of these events and the variety of ways that people interpret and understand these events. In her research, Rust found that bisexual women reported more flux and change in their identities than did lesbians, but they were just as satisfied with their current sexual identities as were lesbians (i.e., they were not confused). Rust describes change as adaptable—bisexual women were able to adjust to changes in their "social landscape" that included sexual and intimate relationships and political affiliations. While the linear models stress stability, Rust stresses adaptability.

Rust's work, my own preliminary studies of identity development, and many discussions with a variety of lesbian, gay, and bisexual people about their experiences with identity formation, led me to reject the linear models. I was convinced that coming out has no set boundaries—no clear beginning and ending points—and that understanding required sensitivity to other interrelated human identities such as gender and race. My model (Eliason, 1996b), which is illustrated in

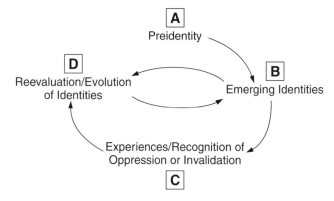

FIGURE 2.2.   The relationship among the cycles of identity formation.

Figure 2.2, can be used to describe any aspect of identity. The model has the following four cycles:

1. *Preidentity.* A person must know that a label or a category of person exists before she/he can adopt an identity. Many lesbian, gay, and bisexual people report feeling different as children, but not knowing what to call that difference until attaining some recognition of the concept of homosexuality. This recognition may come from taunts of other children ("sissy," "fag"), from an attraction to someone of the same sex, from a comment made by a parent, or from some reference to homosexuality in a book or movie, or on TV. The same is true for other identities. For example, children who live in poverty may not be aware of class differences until the media or some event such as taunting (comments such as "white trash" or "wrong side of the tracks") makes it clear that other children live differently. Gender is learned very early in life and even very young children can accurately identify their sex and gender. On the other hand, sexuality is more taboo and children may not be exposed to lesbian, gay, and bisexual options until much later.

2. *Identity Exploration.* Once a label is discovered, the person can try it on and see if it fits. Identity exploration is the most dangerous time of the coming out process, because many people explore their sexuality with very little factual information about safe sex or about safe relationships. Those with internalized homophobia may drown their sorrows in alcohol or drugs or other self-destructive behavior. A

parallel in racial identity development can be found—some young people as they explore a minority racial identity develop a sense of hopelessness or internalized racism. This can be manifest as violence or depression or dejection. Some people successfully negotiate the exploration phase and move on to a healthier position, whereas other people stagnate in the exploration cycle for many years.

3. *Experiences of Discrimination or Invalidation.* In the third cycle, some identities become central to the individual. If a person experiences discrimination directly, observes that others of the same group are discriminated against, or feels that society does not validate her/his identity, that identity may take precedence over others. For example, a bisexual European American man may be accepted by society for his race and gender, but be discriminated against because of his sexual identity. His sense of himself as bisexual may become the most important identity at that point in time. However, the African American lesbian may be invalidated simultaneously for her race, gender, and sexuality, and may not be able to isolate these identities—they are equally important to her. The lack of discrimination faced by White people because of race, and heterosexual people because of sexuality helps to explain why these identities usually remain peripheral ones for them, and why they may have difficulty understanding the importance of racial or sexual identities to others.

4. *Identity Reevaluation.* So much research has indicated that sexuality is fluid that any coming out model must have room for change. Identities can be reevaluated or changed at any time, which may send the person back through another identity exploration cycle. Life circumstances change—new jobs, new economic situations, and new sexual and emotional relationships may all result in identity evolution. This does not imply that all people change their sexual identities on a regular basis. In fact, most people perceive their sexuality as somewhat stable and fixed, but other identities may change or flux more dramatically in ways that affect sexuality.

In this model, the individual identity processes interact with the social world. Figure 2.3 shows how the individual is situated in terms of these other social institutions and relationships—influences which can alter the formation of sexual identity dramatically.

This model assumes that all forms of identity develop according to the same processes—class, gender, racial, and sexual identities form

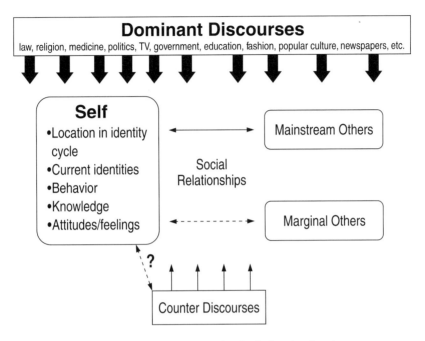

FIGURE 2.3.   Influences on individual identity development.

more or less simultaneously as we grow, but are experienced differently at different points in life and in different social situations. The
value of this cyclical model of coming out is clear: it considers the in-
terconnections of human identities, assumes that change might be
healthy and adaptive, and sees identity formation as a lifelong process
with no clear beginnings or end.

Whether experienced as discrete, linear stages or a gradual cyclical
process, coming out is a positive experience for most lesbian, gay, and
bisexual people. Living with secrets or hiding significant relationships always has negative consequences on self-esteem and mental
health. Feelings of shame, guilt, fear, and/or embarrassment often accompany the secrets of the closet, and coming out is usually associated with relief, increased self-esteem, better health, and even intense
joy. Research has indicated that a positive sense of self as lesbian, gay,
or bisexual is associated with an increased feeling of personal integrity (Rand, Graham, & Rawlings, 1982), increased ability to form
intimate relationships (Cramer & Roach, 1988; Wells & Kline, 1987),

fewer feelings of isolation (Murphy, 1989), a decrease in mental health problems such as depression, social anxiety, and low self-esteem (Miranda & Storms, 1989; Savin-Williams, 1989; Schmitt & Kurdek, 1987) and greater acceptance from others (Olsen, 1987). However, it is not so simple as to just tell lesbian, gay, and bisexual people to come out for their own health. Coming out can still have tremendous negative consequences such as workplace discrimination or loss of job (Hall, 1989; Levine & Leonard, 1984).

Badgett (1996) has developed an economic model to predict coming out in the workplace. She explored many factors that influence that decision to disclose sexual identity to boss or co-workers, including the type of company or organization, whether the company has a policy that prohibits discrimination on the basis of sexual orientation, and factors unique to each individual such as age, health status, relationship status, education, income, race, religion, and degree of outness in other settings. Heterosexual people do not have to consider the possibility of losing their jobs if they "come out" in the workplace or if they talk about their significant others or families at the job. Because they have never considered the possibility, it may be difficult for them to understand how stressful the workplace can be for lesbian, gay, and bisexual people.

Another consequence can be loss of family (Achtenberg, 1988; Falk, 1989). In this regard, sexual identities differ from most other kinds of human identity. If you grow up in a racial minority, your family is generally of the same race as you and remains a steady influence throughout experiences of racism in the world. However, most lesbian, gay, and bisexual people are raised by heterosexual parents, and risk rejection when they come out. Even loving, supportive parents and other family members may experience shock and feelings of grief and loss when a family member comes out (parents' reactions will be described in detail in Chapter 4). In spite of the value our culture puts on honesty, many lesbian, gay, and bisexual people may lose family support for being honest; this is one of the few areas where dishonesty is actively encouraged (consider, also, the military's "don't ask, don't tell" policy). Lesbian, gay, and bisexual people with children risk losing custody of those children as well, a trauma discussed more thoroughly in Chapter 4.

Yet another potential danger of coming out is the risk for discrimination, harassment, and even physical harm (Garnets, Herek, & Levy,

1990; Herek, 1989). Lesbian, gay, and bisexual people are the most targeted group for hate crimes in the United States. Many people, however, are beaten or harassed because someone *perceives* that they are gay, whether they are out or not, so being closeted is not always a protection from discrimination and harassment. Although many therapists and activists strongly recommend coming out because of the mental health benefits, individuals contemplating this action may perceive the risks as being much too high.

Diversity in Lesbian, Gay, and Bisexual Communities

Throughout this book, I refer to lesbian, gay, and bisexual "communities," perhaps implying that there is a well-organized group of people with common goals and a shared philosophy. Unfortunately (or maybe, fortunately), this is not the case. Lesbian, gay, and bisexual people differ on every other human dimension except for their self-imposed sexual identity, and even then, it is not the same to be a lesbian as to be a gay man in our culture, and not the same to be a bisexual woman as to be a bisexual man, or a bisexual man as a gay man, and so on. Important sources of diversity that can also create conflict and divisiveness among lesbian, gay, and bisexual groups include race and ethnicity, socioeconomic class, gender, age, physical abilities or disabilities, urban versus rural residence, and religion. Some of these characteristics will be discussed in the following sections, as they are crucial factors in health and health care.

Racial and Ethnic Diversity

Lesbian, gay, and bisexual people in the United States belong to all the recognized racial groups, representing African American, Latino(a), Asian American, and Native American populations, as well as all ethnicities. Within each racial and ethnic group, there is also considerable diversity. For example, "Asians" includes people from several culturally distinct countries in East and South Asia as well as many Pacific Islands. Many people consider "Jewish" as a race or ethnicity, but for purposes of this chapter, I will include it in the section on religion, although I recognize Jewish cultural differences extend well beyond religious beliefs or practices.

It might seem that a group of people who are oppressed by dominant society, as lesbian, gay, and bisexual people are, would be more tolerant of other kinds of human diversity, or even embrace issues of racial difference. However, European American lesbian, gay, and bisexual people are socialized into the same racist society as everyone else, and they are racist to varying degrees. People of color who hope to find support and friendship in lesbian, gay, and bisexual communities often encounter racism, both in subtle and blatant fashion. The following argument is often heard in lesbian, gay, or bisexual organizations:

The purpose of this group is to promote the needs of people who are oppressed because of their sexuality. If we attend to other issues like race or gender, it will take our energy away from our main goal.

This argument makes people of color (and women, disabled people, Jews, and so on) invisible in these organizations because identities cannot be separated or parceled out. A person of color who is lesbian, gay, or bisexual faces both racism and homophobia on a daily basis, but because of the visibility of racial markers, racism may be the central concern (Chan, 1989; Mays & Cochran, 1986). It can be difficult finding social and political groups that meet the needs of people of color. For example, Audre Lorde (1982) described not finding acceptance in lesbian organizations because of her race (African American), not feeling validated in civil rights groups because of her sexuality (lesbian) or gender (woman), and an outsider in society because of the intersections of all three oppressions. She wisely noted that oppressions cannot be rank ordered or placed on a hierarchy. Racism is not worse than sexism, for example; they are equally bad. And oppressions are not simply additive as in one oppression plus another oppression equals a double oppression. Instead, race, sex, gender, and other forms of oppression interact in often unpredictable ways.

Although European American lesbian, gay, and bisexual people may experience oppression when their sexual identity is known, they also enjoy the privilege and opportunities of their racial identity. White gay and bisexual men enjoy male privilege as well, evidenced by statistics suggesting that White gay males make more money, as a group, than lesbians, bisexual women, or heterosexual White women. Openly gay White men make less money than heterosexual White men, however

(Badgett, 1996). Racism and sexism can have profound economic implications, so that people of color in general make less money than European Americans, and women, as a group, make less money than men. For lesbian, gay, and bisexual people of color, financial difficulties, with all their implications for health, are a major problem.

Some differences that lesbian, gay, and bisexual people of color may have as a group include disclosure decisions, different manifestations of homophobia in their racial communities, and perceptions of conflicting allegiances. European American lesbian, gay, and bisexual political organizations often emphasize coming out as a personal and political strategy. People of color, however, may depend more on their families and racial communities for support from racism and a feeling of cultural comfort, and therefore may choose not to come out (Espín, 1987; Tremble, Schneider, & Appathurai, 1989). European Americans may incorrectly interpret this reluctance to come out to family as a sign of internalized homophobia or lack of commitment to lesbian, gay, or bisexual identity.

Homophobia is as prevalent in racial minority groups as in European American cultures, although the reasons for it may differ somewhat. Some African American heterosexuals view homosexuality as a threat to the survival of black families in much the same ways that interracial marriages are viewed—they chastise African American lesbian, gay, and bisexual people for not propagating the race (ignoring that many do indeed have children), and for their allegiances to predominantly White lesbian, gay, and bisexual organizations (Greene, 1986). Many people of color keenly express the conflicting allegiances between racial and sexual minority social and political communities (Conerly, 1996; Hemphill, 1991; Lee, 1996; Loiacano, 1989; Morales, 1989; Ramos, 1994; Silvera, 1991).

Interracial relationships are another potential source of conflict and stress. Since homosexuality is a statistical minority and people of color are also in the minority in the United States, it may be more difficult for lesbian, gay, or bisexual people of color to find partners within their own racial groups. Interracial relationships can be difficult when the European American partner behaves in racist fashion, does not recognize the profound effects of racism, or denies that race is an issue. The couple may experience social difficulties in all communities (Slater, 1995). For example: "I was ostracized [by a Black lesbian group] for leaving a Black lover and having a relationship with a White woman. I was told I had let the side down and was accused of selling out" (Mason-John & Khambatta, 1993, p. 29).

Another difference between minority and majority lesbian, gay, and bisexual people may lie in the terminology used for self-labeling. Mason-John and Khambatta (1993) suggested that there may be resistance to accepting Western labels among some people of color: "Labelling . . . placing people in rigid categories and imposing a name tag . . . has been a common feature of colonisation . . . in the lesbian and gay world, the terminology which has developed is born out of White western experience" (p. 38).

Most of what we know of the experiences of lesbian, gay, and bisexual people of color comes from anthologies of personal writing and not from empirical research. Why is this? One reason is that the academy continues to be dominated by White heterosexual men, and even gay studies consists mostly of White gay men and a few White lesbians (Duggan, 1992). White people are still struggling with understanding the importance of race and often do not recognize that our research is based on a White perspective—we tend to take White as the norm and try to plug others into a White model (this is also a problem of health care systems that have a Eurocentric bias). Another problem is that people of color often do not volunteer for research studies because of their legitimate fear of being misrepresented or exploited. A potential respondent in Celia Kitzinger's study of lesbianism wrote her this letter:

> . . . torn between the homophobia of the black community and the racism of the white lesbian community, I need, as a black lesbian, to speak for myself and in my own voice, which is not the voice of the white world. I do not want my black experience filtered through your white academic language, the rage and passion edited out, explained away. I do not doubt your good intentions; I do doubt your ability to comprehend or accurately represent my lesbianism, which cannot be taken out of the context of my blackness. (Kitzinger, 1987, p. 88)

In the spirit of the preceding anonymous respondent, the following are experiences of people of color, in their own voices:

> As Latinas, we are supposed to grow up submissive, virtuous, respectful of elders and helpful to our mothers, long suffering,

deferring to men, industrious and devoted. We also know that any deviation from these expectations constitutes an act of rebellion and there is great pressure to conform . . . . Being a lesbian is by definition an act of treason against our cultural values. (Mariana Romo-Carmona, 1987, p. xxvi)

When I speak of home, I mean not only the familial constellation from which I grew, but the entire Black community; the Black press, the Black church, Black academicians, the Black literati, and the Black left. Where is my reflection? I am most often rendered invisible, perceived as a threat to the family, or I am tolerated if I am silent and inconspicuous. I cannot go home as who I am and that hurts me deeply. (Joseph Beam, 1986, p. 231)

Connie Chan (1989) interviewed Asian American lesbian and gay people and found several common themes including the idea that adopting a lesbian or gay identity meant rejecting the most important role for women and men in Asian culture—motherhood and fatherhood. For sons in particular, continuation of the family line was stressed. When asked about the conflict between their Asian and gay identities, respondents had different viewpoints:

I choose gay, because I feel my sexual orientation transcends my Asian American identity. I also feel that I can have a greater impact in changing attitudes in the gay population.

Asian American, because I can't deal with the White-dominated lesbian and gay scene. I guess I'm more race conscious than sexual orientation conscious.

The only identification I can feel comfortable with is one which acknowledges both my lesbian and my Asian-American identities. (all quotes, p. 18)

Makeda Silvera (1990) discussed the conflict in allegiances:

Many lesbians have worked, like me, in the struggles of Black people since the 1960s. We have been on marches every time one of us gets murdered by the police. We have been at sit-ins and vigils. . . . And we have all at one time or another given support to men in our community, all the time painfully holding onto, obscuring our secret lives. When we do walk out of the closet (or are thrown out), the "ideologues" of the Black communities say "Yes, she was a radical sistern but, I don't know what happen, she just went the wrong way." What is implicit in this is that one cannot be a lesbian and continue to do political work (p. 58) . . . . Too often white women focus only on their oppression as lesbians, ignoring the more complex oppression of non-white women who are also lesbians. We remain outsiders in these groups, without images or political voices that echo our own . . . . As Afro-Caribbean women, we are still at the stage where we have to imagine and discover our own existence, past and present. As lesbians, we are even more marginalized, less visible. (p. 59)

Native American cultures differ from the others to some degree, because there is a long tradition of accepting gender and sexual difference, and even of celebrating it. European writers gave the name *berdache* to Native Americans who adopted cross-gender roles in their tribes. Roscoe (1987) found evidence of 133 Native American tribes who had recognized roles for berdache men and/or women or both.

In the old days, during life on the plains, the people respected each other's vision. Berdaches had an integral place in the rigors and lifestyle of the tribe. The way they were viewed was not the same as the contemporary Indian gay lifestyle and consciousness that we have now—they were not fighting for a place in society and to be accepted by that society. They already had a place, a very special and sacred place. They were the people who gave sacred names, cut down the Sun Dance pole, and foretold future events. . . . But all this changed with the coming of the reservation period in Indian history and the systematic crushing of all things Indian. (M. Owlfeather, 1988, p. 100)

Race has a significant impact on health care in the United States, where people of color are disproportionately poor. Lesbian, gay, or bisexual people of color may suffer even more stress than heterosexual people of color, and have less support when they are ill. Racism, sexism, and heterosexism interact in unpredictable and complex ways to complicate the lives of people of color in the United States (Greene, 1994).

Gender

There is ample evidence that women and men differ in many significant ways. There is no consensus as to whether the differences are biologically based, are the result of differential socialization, or are caused by some interaction of the two, but undoubtedly sexism is alive and well. Women make less money than men, are less likely to be promoted to higher positions, are more often victims of sexual assault, and are still disproportionately found in the nurturing professions such as nursing, social work, and teaching, which are underpaid and undervalued. Lesbian and bisexual women differ from gay and bisexual men in these same ways, and also in personality patterns that have demonstrated gender differences, such as emphasis on relationships versus individual rights, aggression, attitudes about casual sex, motives for sex, need for intimacy, and so on. These fundamental differences may create conflict in lesbian, gay, and bisexual political and social groups.

For example, gay men often report sexual activity with men before adopting a gay identity; sex is one of the ways that a gay identity is achieved (Herdt, 1989; Paroski, 1987; Weinberg, 1978), whereas lesbians are more likely to experience intimate and emotional connections to women before having any sexual attractions (Gramick, 1984; Sears, 1989). Like heterosexual men, gay men are more likely to choose partners initially on the basis of physical attractiveness or sexual desirability, with the hopes that love may follow, whereas lesbians, like heterosexual women, are more likely to seek love and romance from the beginning (Blumstein & Schwartz, 1983; Wilson, 1987).

Gay men are more likely to view their sexuality as inborn or genetic and to define themselves by their sexual difference (Hencken, 1984), and lesbians are more likely as a group to give a broad range of explanations that include biology, affectional preferences and choices, and political choices (Eliason & Morgan, 1996a; Hunnisett, 1986). Lesbians often define themselves in terms beyond sexual difference (Faderman, 1984; Ponse, 1984). A 32-year-old European-American lesbian described herself as follows: "Being a lesbian is essential to my identity, my sense of self, my politics and many of my social support choices—and increasingly integrated into my work/career as an active out lesbian-identified professional" (Eliason & Morgan, 1996a).

Gender differences may cause as many conflicts and lead to as many misunderstandings between lesbian and bisexual women and gay and bisexual men as they do between heterosexual women and men.

Class

Socioeconomic class is a major factor in health care. People from the working or underclasses have variable access to health care, and the care they receive may be of poor quality. Class differences found in mainstream society, with its strong classist attitudes, are also found in lesbian, gay, and bisexual communities. Sexual minorities come from every class background.

We do not discuss class issues often in our culture, partly because no one can clearly define class, partly because we tend to believe the myth that all people are equally able to "pull themselves up by their bootstraps," and because the topic makes many people uncomfortable. Pauline Bart (1994) defined class as follows:

Class is multidimensional. It's not just about money—it's about power and prestige and self-concept and self-image and "lifestyle" and whether you can get your teeth straightened or your nose straightened . . . and whether you want to do so. (p. 4)

Within standard middle-class norms, the myth prevails that if you work hard you will get ahead, even though many economic indicators argue against it. But many working-class lesbians have no such illusions:

I never bought in to the American myth about working hard and making it. I knew no one could work any harder than my parents, and making it meant survival. There are others who work hard and don't survive. My Mom has health insurance. Many do not. (McMichael, 1994, p. 340)

A popular myth perpetuated by radical right wing organizations is that lesbian, gay, and bisexual people are wealthy and powerful enough to force their "gay agenda" onto the U.S. political scene. The truth is that lesbian, gay, and bisexual people are distributed by income levels in much the same way that heterosexuals are—a few are wealthy, many are middle class, and a significant number are working poor, or destitute or homeless.

Age

We live in a youth-oriented culture. You need only to watch the most popular television shows, view a few minutes of MTV, or look at the ads in most magazines to see the truth of that statement. Advertisements implore us to cover that gray hair, smooth out those age wrinkles, or have costly and dangerous surgery to alter the aging process in our bodies. When lesbian, gay, or bisexual people are depicted in the media, they are almost always young adults. Most lesbian, gay, and bisexual organizations are youth oriented as well, with activities such as rallies, parades, and dances that cater to young people. Middle-aged and older adult lesbian, gay, and bisexual people are largely invisible in society as well as in lesbian, gay, and bisexual organizations, and little is known about the unique issues they may have. Older adults are also much more likely to experience health problems that force them to deal with health care systems where they experience ageism and their sexuality is denied (old people are not supposed to be sexual beings). I will discuss unique problems of older lesbian, gay, and bisexual people in Chapter 6.

Religion

Lesbian, gay, and bisexual people also come from every possible type of religious or spiritual background. Since the United States is still predominantly Judeo-Christian, the following discussion focuses on the Christian and Jewish religions. Most of Judeo-Christian doctrine is based on various interpretations of the Bible, and it has become a major source of antigay rhetoric in the United States. However, as I will discuss in the following chapter, the Bible actually has very little to say about homosexuality, and some of the passages used to condemn homosexuality may have been misinterpreted or taken out of context. Nevertheless, many Christian denominations have accepted antigay bias as God's word, and consider homosexuality to be a sin. Lesbian, gay, and bisexual people who grow up in these religions must make choices: give up their religion for their mental health, remain closeted in their churches and experience self-hatred and condemnation, find a more accepting religion, or resolve spiritual issues on a personal level without a congregation. Mel White, formerly a minister for the Christian Right and ghostwriter of biographies of Pat Robertson and Jerry Falwell, was ostracized by his former friends when he came out as a Christian gay man. White continues to have strong faith and preach God's acceptance, not God's condemnation, while leading the battle against antigay religious teachings.

Jewish lesbian, gay, and bisexual people face anti-Semitism from the heterosexual Christian world, as well as from gentile lesbian, gay, and bisexual people. Warren Blumenfeld (1996) noted the similarities between anti-Semitism and homophobia by comparing the ways that Jews and homosexuals both have been depicted as morally weak, carriers of disease, and violators of gender roles. These parallels were noted in Nazi Germany propaganda as well as in the White supremacist and Christian Right propaganda of today. Again, despite the similarities of homophobia and anti-Semitism, many lesbian, gay, and bisexual people are unaware of anti-Semitism. For example:

> *Repeatedly, I find that I am preoccupied not with countering anti-Semitism, but with trying to prove that anti-Semitism exists, that it is serious, and that, as lesbian/feminists, we should be paying attention to it both inside and outside the movement . . . the anti-Semitism with which I am immediately concerned, and which I find most threatening does not take the form of the overt undeniably inexcusable painted Swastika on a Jewish gravestone or on a synagogue wall. Instead, it is elusive and difficult to pinpoint, for it is the anti-Semitism either of omission or one which trivializes Jewish experience and Jewish oppression. (Klepfisz, 1982, p. 46)*

Traditional Jewish law does not mention lesbians, making a Jewish lesbian an enigma in her community. Evelyn Torton Beck (1982, p. xv) noted, "If I say that Judaism is more than a religion, as lesbianism is more than a sexual preference, I begin to tap the complexity." Both identities can have profound effects on both a person's sense of self and the way that she/he is treated by others.

Political Involvement

The stereotypical image of the "gay person" is an angry young man waving a protest sign or cavorting in a gay pride parade—a political and cultural radical. The truth is that some lesbian, gay, and bisexual people are not political at all, whereas others have conservative, liberal, or socialist views. Like most Americans, lesbian, gay, and bisexual people are not very involved in politics—they probably vote in about the same numbers as heterosexual people and very few belong to the highly visible political action groups such as Queer Nation or ACT-UP, or indeed any group based on sexual identity. However, demonstrations and gay pride parades make news, and thus perpetuate stereotypes. Attending a gay pride rally does not really constitute a political act for many of the participants, but rather an opportunity for socializing. For a few, it is a truly political act.

Whenever I do a workshop on lesbian, gay, and bisexual issues, someone inevitably asks: "Why must you people have those parades and rallies? Heterosexuals don't have straight pride rallies." There are several reasons gay pride celebrations are important and a necessary part of gay life today. First, lesbian, gay, and bisexual people often feel isolated and alone in their neighborhoods, places of employment, classes, and churches. A yearly gay pride event allows them to come together and celebrate their lives. For a few hours, they can be in the majority instead of being a hated minority. Second, heterosexual people can affirm their identities in myriad ways: by putting engagement, wedding, birth, and anniversary announcements in the newspaper, by bringing their families to work-related social events, and by having family reunions. Lesbian, gay, and bisexual people often lack that support, and need to create their own ways of affirming themselves. Gay pride parades are one way . . . and heterosexuals also have parades—homecoming, Mardi Gras, wedding dances, the Tournament of Roses parade, and many other kinds of celebrations all affirm heterosexuality.

Origins or "Causes" of Sexual Orientation

I have enclosed the word causes in this section title in quotation marks because we rarely ask about the cause of heterosexuality. Why then is our culture obsessed with the cause of homosexuality or bisexuality? For many lesbian, gay, and bisexual people, the cause of their sexuality is not of concern—they are more interested in being accepted for who they are and ending discrimination than in finding a cause. Since our culture is obsessed with the causes, however, I will briefly address the range of theories that have been advanced to explain lesbian, gay, and bisexual sexual orientations. These theories can generally be categorized as biologically based or environmental. I will review only more recent "scientific" studies here; some of the older "unscientific" theories that explained homosexuality as "sin" or "crimes against nature" continue to influence attitudes but are rarely expressed in the scientific literature. All of the following theories take heterosexuality for granted as the "normal" sexuality. Very little time has been devoted to the study of heterosexual identity per se.

Biologically Based Theories

There are some fairly strong arguments for the biological basis of sexual orientation. Across very different cultures in the world, the rate of homosexuality and bisexuality is fairly consistent (Diamond, 1993). If cultural or social factors caused sexual orientation, this consistency would be unlikely. Recent research on biological origins of sexuality falls into two categories: genetics and prenatal hormonal exposure. Both sets of theories assume that the genetic or hormonal mechanism can result in brain differences in homosexuals and heterosexuals that are presumed to cause sexual differences.

Genetic theories gained credence after several published reports of twin studies, in which monozygotic twins were found to have a higher concordance for homosexuality than dizygotic twin pairs or other siblings (e.g., Bailey & Pillard, 1991; Whitam, Diamond, & Martin, 1993). In a study that made headlines in major newspapers across the country, researchers conducted DNA linkage analyses for 40 families that had two gay brothers (Homer, Hu, Magnuson, Hu, & Pattatucci, 1993). They found a genetic marker on the X chromosome (Xp28) in common in 64% of the cases. Obviously, this study cannot explain all of homosexuality—only males were studied and 36% of the cases could not be explained by the genetic marker. Nor does the study attempt to explain bisexuality. But the headlines generally read: "Homosexuality Is Genetic."

Another news-making headline came earlier, in 1991, from research conducted by Simon LeVay. He studied brain tissue from 41 deceased individuals; 19 were gay men who had died of AIDS, 16 were presumably heterosexual men who had died of other causes, and 6 were presumably heterosexual women who had died of causes other than AIDS.

On microscopic exam, LeVay found a small area of the hypothalamus (one of the interstitial nuclei of the anterior hypothalamus: INAH3) was twice as large in heterosexual men than in gay men or heterosexual women. This study has some obvious problems: The sample was small, the gay men died of AIDS, which is known to affect the brain; the sexual identity of the other subjects was only presumed to be heterosexual, but not confirmed; and the area of difference was so small that the measurements may not be reliable. And again, lesbians and bisexuals of either sex were not studied.

The prenatal hormonal theories are based on the assumption that something goes awry in prenatal life—the mother is exposed to some substance, or is under stress, which causes her body to release abnormal levels of sex hormones that alter the course of fetal development. Animal research suggests that providing the "wrong" sex hormone in prenatal life can alter brain development in the areas controlling sexual drives, so that the "feminized" male will exhibit female sexual behaviors, such as submission, and the "masculinized" female will mount other animals (see Hamer & Copeland, 1994; Schmidt & Clement, 1995, for a review of these studies). These studies, though widely cited, have one significant flaw—animals are not people, and sexual behavior is much more complex in humans than in animals who are driven by an estrus cycle.

DeCecco and Parker (1995) have suggested that all the biological explanations for homosexuality are based on five underlying assumptions:

1. Sexual behavior is determined by biology, not learned.
2. Homosexuality and heterosexuality are entirely different phenomena, not on a continuum.
3. Homosexuality is associated with "feminine" traits in gay men, and with "masculine" traits in lesbians.
4. Finding that homosexuality is biological will result in improved attitudes and less discrimination.
5. Biology is a value-free, objective science.

DeCecco and Parker noted that none of these assumptions have been proven to be true, and they advocate a more broad-based approach to the study of sexuality that incorporates a bio-psycho-social-cultural model.

Environmental Theories

The environmental theories include a wide range of ideas about the origins of lesbian, gay, or bisexual identities. The older environmental theories tended to blame parents for their children's sexuality. Psychoanalytic theories often proposed that a clinging, overprotective mother with a distant, absent father created the male homosexual, who identified with his mother rather than his father. Other theories blamed mothers for giving their boys mixed messages about gender (e.g., dressing them in frills or giving them dolls). The following are among the other proposed theories:

- Girls who were sexually abused by men would grow up to be lesbians because they fear or hate men.
- Boys who were sexually abused by men would develop a yearning for male-male sex as adults.
- Homosexuality is a character defect.
- Homosexuality is rejection of societal gender roles.
- Lack of resolution of the Oedipal complex can cause homosexuality.
- Homosexuality represents masculine protest (in compensation for women's inferiority).
- All people are born bisexual and have masculine and feminine traits.
- Seduction by an older lesbian, gay, or bisexual person while the child is at an impressionable age leads to homosexuality.

There is no strong support for any of these environmental theories (Bell & Weinberg, 1978), nor can the biological theories explain all instances of homosexuality or bisexuality. It appears likely either that sexual orientation is determined by a biology-environment interaction (as suggested by DeCecco & Parker, 1995), or that there are multiple paths to forming a sexual identity—for some people, sexuality is driven by genetic or other biological factors; and for others, sexuality is determined by personal, cultural, or social factors. Heterosexuality may also be multiply determined.

CONCLUSION

In this chapter, I have reviewed some basic information about lesbian, gay, and bisexual people, beginning with a brief historical overview. Homophobia and heterosexism were discussed as well as the coming out process by which people achieve a sexual identity. Health care professionals need to understand these concepts, which can have direct influence on health. The forms of diversity within lesbian, gay, and bisexual communities also are important determinants of health and of access to health care. The chapter concluded with a discussion of the possible origins of sexual orientation.

EXERCISE: AM I HOMOPHOBIC?

This activity measures your own level of homophobia. The following items constitute the Index of Homophobia developed by Hudson and Ricketts in 1980. Read each item and assign a rating of 1 to 5 where:

1 = Strongly Agree   3 = Don't Know   5 = Strongly Disagree
2 = Agree   4 = Disagree

_____ a. I would feel comfortable working closely with a male homosexual.
_____ b. I would enjoy attending social functions at which homosexuals were present.
_____ c. I would feel uncomfortable if I learned that my neighbor was homosexual.
_____ d. If a member of my sex made a sexual advance toward me, I would feel angry.
_____ e. I would feel comfortable knowing that I was attractive to members of my sex.
_____ f. I would feel uncomfortable being seen in a gay bar.
_____ g. I would feel comfortable if a member of my sex made an advance toward me.
_____ h. I would feel comfortable if I found myself attracted to a member of my sex.

_____ i. I would feel disappointed if I learned that my child was homosexual.

_____ j. I would feel nervous being in a group of homosexuals.

_____ k. I would feel comfortable knowing that my clergy was homosexual.

_____ l. I would be upset if I learned that my brother or sister was homosexual.

_____ m. I would feel that I had failed as a parent if I learned that my child was gay.

_____ n. If I saw two men holding hands in public, I would feel disgusted.

_____ o. If a member of my sex made an advance toward me, I would feel offended.

_____ p. I would feel comfortable if I learned that my daughter's teacher was a lesbian.

_____ q. I would feel uncomfortable if I learned that my spouse/partner was attracted to his/her own sex.

_____ r. I would feel at ease talking with a homosexual person at a party.

_____ s. I would feel uncomfortable if I learned that my boss was a homosexual.

_____ t. It would not bother me to walk through a predominantly gay section of town.

_____ u. It would disturb me to find out that my doctor was homosexual.

_____ v. I would feel comfortable if I learned that my best friend of my sex was homosexual.

_____ w. If a member of my sex made an advance toward me, I would feel flattered.

_____ x. I would feel uncomfortable knowing that my son's teacher was a male homosexual.

_____ y. I would feel uncomfortable working closely with a lesbian.

To score the scale, reverse-score half of the items: Change a 1 to a 5, a 2 to a 4, leave 3's as they are, change a 4 to a 2, and change a 5 to a 1 for the following items—c, d, f, i, j, l, m, n, o, q, s, u, x, and y. Now add up your score, and subtract 25. This is your homophobia score. Hudson and Ricketts provided the following guidelines for interpreting the score:

0-25   = nonhomophobic
26-50   = mildly homophobic
51-75   = moderately homophobic
76-100   = extremely homophobic

In a recent study of heterosexual university employees (Eliason & Raheim, in press), we found that 15% of the respondents were nonhomophobic, 39% were mildly homophobic, 33% were moderately homophobic, and 13% were extremely homophobic.

You might also want to look at individual items. If some of the items made you feel more uncomfortable than others, think about why. Are you more comfortable with the thought of dealing with lesbian, gay, or bisexual strangers, such as people at a party or in the workplace, than you are with the thought of having a lesbian, gay, or bisexual family member or close friend? These items may give you some insight into your own feelings.

CHAPTER THREE

The Damage Done by Negative Stereotypes

I SEE MYSELF AS A black person first, then as a deaf person, and then as a gay person . . . since my skin color is visible, they can identify me as black. Then they find out I'm deaf. As for being gay, it's a sticky situation. I'm not really in the closet, but I have to use my best judgment to trust people to accept me as a gay person. That is the last thing, yet the main concern of all my identities is my gayness. ("Pablo" 1993, p. 39)

In this chapter, I will discuss some common stereotypes that plague lesbian, gay, and bisexual people, and counter these beliefs with accurate information based on empirical research. Stereotypes are generalized ideas that are applied to all members of a group, such as women are nurturing and men are aggressive. (In reality, many men are nurturers and women are quite capable of aggression.) Stereotypes can be positive, negative, or neutral, but are always damaging to individuals within the group by denying them their unique humanity. Negative attitudes about homosexuality and bisexuality are fueled and maintained by stereotypes. By far the most damaging and pervasive myths have to do with the role of religion. How often have you heard someone say, "Homosexuality is a sin," or "The Bible says it's wrong"? Most people who make these statements cannot explain what they mean or cite the actual source of their beliefs. Because of the confusion regarding religion and homosexuality, I will devote a significant portion of this chapter to what the Bible actually says, and will explore some of the current changes in the position being taken by many religious denominations.

In the remainder of the chapter, I will explore stereotypes based on gender—the myth that gay men are more like women and lesbians are more like men and the related myth that you can identify lesbian, gay, or bisexual people by their gender-atypical appearance, behavior, or occupation; that homosexuality is caused by a bad experience with someone of the same sex; that homosexuals are child molesters or "recruit" unsuspecting heterosexuals; and that same-sex relationships are unstable. I will also look at myths about changing sexual identity, stereotypes related to sexual practices, myths about HIV and AIDS, and some unique stereotypes about bisexuals.

The quote that begins this chapter is a reminder that many lesbian, gay, and bisexual people have multiple identities. Sexual identity intersects with other human identities, some of which may also be marginalized. The experiences of a deaf gay African American man will be different from the experiences of a hearing lesbian Asian American or a physically disabled Native American bisexual man.

Doesn't the Bible Condemn Homosexuality?

Religion plays a major role in attitudes about sexuality in our culture, as evidenced by the current debates about abortion, birth control, unwed mothers, and premarital sex. Fundamentalist Christian groups, in particular, often use religion to justify negative attitudes about lesbian, gay, and bisexual people although not all religions or religious leaders agree on these issues. In my discussion, I will focus on Judeo-Christian doctrines, since they are the most pervasive in the United States.

Members of many churches cite the Bible to justify antigay sentiment but rarely can identify exactly what the Bible says about it. They may take passages out of context or select some passages and ignore others. In addition, the Bible has been translated many times, and each edition has been influenced by the attitudes of the translators. There are only six brief passages in the Bible that can be interpreted as concerning same-sex sexuality (remember that the concept of a homosexual person did not exist during the period when the Bible was written). Because these passages have been widely cited, I will examine most of them in some detail; first, however, we should remember that people read the Bible in two main ways: either literally, accepting every word as the absolute truth; or historically-critically, which means interpreting words and ideas based on their historical context.

If you were to accept Bible as literal truth, you would have to advocate slavery (e.g., Ephesians 6:5–9; Colossians 3:22–4:1; 1 Timothy 6:1–2). You would have to accept cutting off your hands or gouging out your eyes as a remedy for temptation (Matthew 5:22–29). You would have to believe that women cannot speak in church (1 Timothy 2:11–14), or wear gold jewelry or pearls, or bare their heads in church (1 Timothy 2:9–10; 1 Corinthians 11:1–16). Very few people are willing to accept all of the Bible as absolute truth, so this discussion of the Bible will take the historical-critical approach.

The verse in the Bible most often cited as evidence of God's condemnation of homosexuality is Leviticus 18:22, "You shall not lie with a male as with a woman; it is an abomination," or its companion verse, Leviticus 20:13, "If a man lies with a male as with a woman, both of them have committed an abomination; they shall be put to death, their blood is upon them." This sounds very serious: The offense warrants a death penalty. However, Leviticus also demands death for those who curse their parents, have sex with a menstruating woman, eat pork, lobsters, or shrimp, sow two kinds of grain in the same field, or commit adultery. Leviticus 18:22 and 20:13 are passages embedded within the "Holiness Code," a set of prescriptions for behavior that were intended to set the Israelites apart from gentiles by creating a race of people who were holy or close to God.

Terminology also changes over time. We consider the word *abomination* to be a very strong term, or to refer to something absolutely unacceptable. In Biblical times, however, it was just another word for "unclean." If something was unclean, or an abomination, it meant you needed to "clean up your act." Many current Bible scholars believe that male homosexual acts were fairly common in Canaanite fertility rites at the time, and that the Holiness Code forbade them primarily because Canaanites, who were considered "unclean," engaged in them. Leviticus does not refer to sex between women at all.

The story of Sodom and Gomorrah (Genesis 19:1–11) is also frequently applied to homosexuality. The story goes like this: Two angels in the guise of human beings came to the town of Sodom one day and encountered Lot, who offered them space for the night. He had a feast prepared for the strangers, but soon the men of Sodom surrounded the house, demanding to know who the men were and to "Bring them out to us, so that we may know them." Lot, trying to appease the mob, offered his two virgin daughters to the crowd ("do to them as you please") in return for leaving the strangers alone. The angels struck the men with blindness so that they could not find Lot's door, then advised Lot and his family to leave town because God was going to destroy Sodom and the neighboring town of Gomorrah with fire and brimstone. As they fled, Lot's wife disobeyed the angels' orders and looked back, and was turned into a pillar of salt (often cited as another example of women's unworthiness).

Because the sin of Sodom was interpreted by some people as male homosexual acts, the term "sodomite" came to refer to someone who engages in anal sex. This interpretation comes from the term "to know" which in some Biblical contexts means "to have sex with." Out of 943 uses of forms of "to know" in the Old Testament, only 10 cases (including this one) probably refer to sex. It is possible that the men wanted knowledge of the strangers. Even if they did want sex, the story may be condemning inhospitality and the threat of rape, which in Biblical times (as now) was seen as a means of control and humiliation. Male prisoners of war were often raped or treated like the "inferior" women. Thus, because the men of Sodom were brutal rapists God destroyed the city. The Bible itself supports an interpretation of the Sodom story as the sin of inhospitality. Ezekial 116:48–49 states, "This was the guilt of your sister Sodom: she and her daughters had pride, surfeit of food and prosperous ease, but did not aid the poor and needy." Wisdom 19:13 states that the sin of Sodom was "a bitter hatred of strangers." And modern readers of this story should be appalled by Lot's offering of his daughters to the angry mob, but this is rarely expressed. How could a holy man like Lot be accused of child abuse?

Another passage that is often cited as evidence of condemnation of homosexuality is 1 Corinthians 6:9: "Do not be deceived: neither the immoral, nor idolaters, nor adulterers, nor *(oute malakoi oute arsenokoitai),* nor thieves, nor the greedy, nor drunkards, nor revilers, nor robbers will inherit the kingdom of God." The term *arsenokoitai* in the original text has been translated as "homosexual" (1952 Revised Standard version), "sexual perverts" (1977 Revised Standard), and "male prostitutes and sodomites" (1989 Revised Standard). Other versions of the Bible have translated this word as "child molesters" and "people of infamous habits." This Greek word can be translated literally as men, or male (arseno), and bedroom, bed, or "lying with" (koitai). The word has been used in other contexts to refer to the active partner in sexual intercourse. When the two parts of the word are put together, the meaning is unclear—it could refer to a man who has sex (of any kind), or a man who has sex with other men.

Romans 1:26 is the only passage in the Bible that can be interpreted to condemn female homosexuality, "Their women exchanged natural intercourse for unnatural." So many things were considered "unnatural," however, that the passage could refer to having sex with an uncircumcised man, anal or oral sex, masturbation, or having sex during menstruation.

Most of this discussion of the Bible was drawn from Daniel Helminiak's book, *What the Bible Really Says about Homosexuality* (1994). Interested readers should consult this highly readable text, or other recent, more scholarly books such as John Boswell's *Christianity, Social Tolerance, and Homosexuality* (1980) or his *Same-Sex Unions in Premodern Europe* (1994); Robin Scrogg's *Homosexuality in the New Testament: Contextual Background for Contemporary Debate* (1983); and L. William Countryman's *Dirt, Greed, and Sex: Sexual Ethics in the New Testament and Their Implications for Today* (1988).

Most Christian religious denominations in the United States base their philosophy on the teachings of Jesus found in the New Testament. Jesus had absolutely nothing negative to say about same-sex sexuality; he gathered prostitutes and other sinners around him, preached acceptance, and warned his followers not to judge others. Because of this emphasis on nonviolent, nonjudgmental New Testament scripture, many Christian denominations have revised their church policies and doctrines in recent years, or are currently engaged in debates about sexuality. Only a small number continue actively to condemn homosexuality, predominantly those denominations that advocate a literal interpretation of the Bible. Other denominations welcome lesbian, gay, and bisexual members to their congregations, and a few ordain openly gay, lesbian, or bisexual people to positions of leadership. Some churches offer ceremonies that bless same-sex unions. Many lesbian, gay, and bisexual people are active in church life, but recent changes in society as well as within religion have meant that more can be open and honest within their congregations and worship with their significant others.

Other lesbian, gay, and bisexual people who were raised in mainstream religions that condemned them have turned away from those affiliations. Some banded together to form the Metropolitan Church of Christ, a nondenominational lesbian, gay, and bisexual church that now has congregations in most large cities. Others have bitter feelings about the religions that rejected them when they needed support. To avoid painful confrontations in times of great stress, health care providers should be aware of the religious affiliations and/or wishes of their lesbian, gay, and bisexual clients, as well as the attitudes of hospital chaplains.

Aren't Homosexuals Confused about Their Sex or Gender?

Sex, sexuality, and gender are confusing, overlapping concepts. In the late 1800s, when sexologists first began to label and study sexual identity, the idea of the *sexual invert* was born. This notion that women are biologically programmed to be attracted to men, and that men are hardwired to be attracted to women is based on the assumption that sex determines both gender and sexual identity. Therefore, a man who is attracted to men must have inverted sex and gender making him more like a woman in his sexual desires and appearance. This idea of inversion carried over to personality traits, so that many early sexologists described the womanly appearance and temperament of the gay man, and the "mannish" lesbian. No one studied bisexuals at that time; sexuality was reduced to an either/or proposition—heterosexual or homosexual.

The two volumes of George Henry's *Sex Variants* (1948) are a good example of this assumption of sex determining sexual identity. Dr. Henry was part of an interdisciplinary team of professionals known as the Committee for the Study of Sex Variants in New York City in the 1930s. The goals of the Committee were to identify, treat, and prevent "sex variants," as they called homosexuals. The volume on lesbians describes in great detail the physical and psychological characteristics of the 40 women—all self-identified lesbians—who volunteered for the study. The Committee, who believed that lesbians must be "masculine," recategorized many of the women if they found any signs of femininity; thus, 9 lesbians were described as "narcissistics," 17 as bisexuals, and only 14 as "real" lesbians. Despite their inability to define a real lesbian, or find any distinguishing physical or psychological characteristics, the Committee concluded that lesbians had "an immature form of skeletal development" (defined as broad shoulders and narrow hips), enlarged clitoris, and strong sexual urges. They had no heterosexual control group. Henry's study is typical of much of the literature on homosexuality in the early to mid-twentieth century (see Terry, 1990).

From this concept of the sexual invert comes the stereotype that lesbians or gay men can be identified by their personality, appearance, occupational choices, or behaviors. The stereotypical lesbian is "masculine," with short hair and a stocky muscular build; she talks "rough," swaggers, and wears her keys on a long chain. She works in construction, drives a truck, or operates heavy machinery. The stereotypical gay man is sensitive, caring, good-looking, and immaculately dressed; he is "effeminate" and is an interior decorator, hairdresser, or flight attendant.

Is there any basis to the stereotype about gender atypicality in lesbian, gay, and bisexual people? As is usually the case, stereotypes contain a grain of truth—they do apply to a subset of people in the group. Grellert, Newcomb, and Bentler (1982) compared adult lesbians and gay men (198 of each) to a matched sample of heterosexual women and men (198 of each), on their memories of childhood play activities. The majority of lesbians and gay men reported some degree of cross-sex play activities. Activities that could be categorized as Feminine Play (dolls, dressing up) distinguished heterosexual women from heterosexual men, gay men from heterosexual men, and lesbians from heterosexual women. A category labeled Sports was equally successful in distinguishing among groups, although girls are allowed more freedom in play activities in childhood and tomboys do not necessarily grow up to be lesbians or bisexual women as often as "sissy boys" grow up to be gay or bisexual men.

Among heterosexual men, there is a tendency to become more androgynous over time, allowing a greater range of expression as men age. Gay men were not found to differ by sex-role behaviors across age, presumably because gay men are better able to blend masculine and feminine traits at an early age (Robinson, Skeen, & Flake-Hobson, 1982). The research on gender-related personality traits shows that gay men are more like heterosexual men than they are like lesbians or heterosexual women. Lesbians are more like heterosexual women than men of any sexual identity. The section on gender in Chapter 2 briefly discusses major gender differences.

Lynch and Reilly (1985/1986) examined whether lesbian couples divided household tasks along traditional gender lines; that is, does one member of the couple assume the "masculine" role and the other the "feminine" role? Seventy lesbian couples who had been together for at least one year responded to the questionnaire. The authors found equal sharing of finances, decision making, and household responsibilities. The only area of inequality was in the initiation of sex—one partner usually initiated sex more often than the other. There was no evidence of heterosexual gender role playing in these lesbian couples.

All people are diverse. Some heterosexual men are "sensitive and artistic," some gay men are football players. Some lesbians wear high heels and some heterosexual women are bricklayers. Some heterosexual men are hairdressers and some bisexual men have no fashion sense. Lesbian, gay, and bisexual people can be found engaging in every human career, but a few options are somewhat "safer" havens, such as entertainment and the arts and some human service professions. These fields tend to value diversity or, at least, are more tolerant of human difference. In these more accepting environments, all people have more freedom to express their unique traits. Consider, for example, the androgyny of many male performers in the music industry (Michael Jackson, the artist formerly known as Prince, Little Richard), as well as the number of known lesbian, gay, and bisexual mainstream performers (Elton John, Melissa Etheridge, David Bowie, Mick Jagger, k.d. lang).

It is easy to reinforce stereotypes but difficult to disprove them. When people see a heterosexual woman with no makeup and short hair they tab her as an exception, or don't think about it at all. When they observe a lesbian with no makeup and short hair, they think, "Ah ha! Lesbians have short hair and wear no makeup," and the stereotype is reinforced. And enough lesbian, gay, and bisexual people do dress or act in gender-atypical ways to keep this stereotype alive and well.

HOMOSEXUALITY IS CAUSED BY A BAD EXPERIENCE WITH THE OPPOSITE SEX

Most of the research exploring the influence of early sexual experiences in determining sexual identity has been done on women. When data in the 1970s revealed the high rate of childhood sexual abuse experiences in women, some theorists speculated that these early traumatic experiences might turn women away from adult heterosexual relationships. Indeed, some studies have found that women with rape histories are more likely to have had sexual experiences with women (Belcastro, 1982;

Cohen, 1983; Gundlack & Reiss, 1967; Simari & Baskin, 1982), and that lesbians have had a somewhat higher frequency of incest experiences (Meiselman, 1978; Peretti & Banks, 1984). At least two of these studies, however, found a high rate of "heterosexual aversion" which may be a different phenomenon than lesbianism per se. And many of these studies focus on clinical groups, or are methodologically shaky.

Brannock and Chapman (1990) surveyed 50 matched nonclinical pairs of heterosexual women and lesbians and found no differences on any kind of sexual abuse history. They also found that the lesbians in their sample began to question their sexuality because of sexual and/or emotional attractions to women, not because of any aversion to men.

Peters and Cantrell (1991) surveyed a nonclinical sample of 134 lesbians and 105 heterosexual women (mean age 30 years). Women of both sexual identities had a wide range of childhood sexual experiences, mostly with other children, and primarily with boys. Lesbians reported more positive reactions to these early peer experiences than did heterosexual women. However, early sexual experiences with adults were likely to be rated negatively by heterosexual women (80%) and lesbians (100%); in all cases, the adult was a male. Twenty percent of the heterosexual women and 15% of the lesbians reported intercourse with an adult male before they were age 12. They had about the same rate of incest experiences after the age of 12—13% of the heterosexual women and 17% of the lesbians, and all women reported a negative reaction to this experience now. The lesbian group had experienced more incidents of coerced or forced sexual experiences after the age of 12 than did heterosexual women (67% compared with 28%). However, discriminant function analyses revealed that childhood sexual experiences were not a significant predictor of adult sexual identity.

Isn't There a Link between Homosexuality and Child Molestation?

Old stereotypes of the homosexual were of a shadowy male figure lurking on playgrounds or in locker rooms trying to lure innocent young boys into a "perverted lifestyle." This myth has been particularly damaging—it has resulted in lesbian, gay, and bisexual teachers, scout leaders, coaches and day-care workers losing jobs, or living in fear of discovery. In 1994, a high school teacher from St. Louis was put on probation after revealing his sexual identity in class. He was describing the system of patches that Nazis used to label prisoners in the concentration camps, pointed to the pink triangle and remarked, "As a gay man, I would have been forced to wear one of these." In spite of his popularity among students and his excellent teaching record, this incident led to his release.

This stereotype about child molestation and lesbian, gay, and bisexual people as a bad influence on children has also led to lesbian, gay, and bisexual parents losing custody of their own children. The facts on this matter are unequivocal—children are at much greater risk for sexual abuse from their heterosexual male teachers, their fathers, stepfathers, and older brothers. The vast majority of perpetrators of childhood sexual abuse (over 90%) are heterosexual men (Feierman, 1990; Hall, 1978; Riley, 1975). The other 10% or so include a mix of gay or bisexual men, heterosexual women, and lesbian and bisexual women. In fact, Jenny, Roseler, and Poyer (1994) reported that a child is 100 times more likely to be molested by a heterosexual than by a homosexual.

Part of the confusion lies in the patterns of sexual abuse. Most *pedophiles* (the name given to perpetrators of child sexual abuse) are sexually attracted to children or young adolescents, and gender may not be important. In other cases, sexual abuse is used to control others or to punish wives. Many people assume that an adult man who abuses a little boy or adolescent male must be gay; most pedophiles, however, are heterosexual in their adult sex lives and many are married. On the other hand, the vast majority of lesbian, gay, and bisexual people have sexual relationships only with other consenting adults, not children.

Another misconception is that some of the pedophile organizations, such as the North American Man-Boy Love Association (NAMBLA), are gay organizations. They are not, and most lesbian, gay, and bisexual people condemn child molestation, as do most heterosexuals.

HOMOSEXUAL RELATIONSHIPS DON'T LAST

There are myths that lesbian, gay, and bisexual people are emotionally unstable or mentally ill, or that they are promiscuous, leading to the stereotype that intimate, loving, long-term same-sex relationships are not possible. Part of the myth is true—many relationships don't last, but this is a human problem and not related to sexual identity. The divorce rate for heterosexuals is close to 50% in the United States, yet people seldom condemn heterosexuality for its instability. It is difficult to speculate about whether lesbian, gay, and bisexual people have more frequent, short-term relationships than heterosexuals, because same-sex couples cannot marry. Therefore, there is nothing comparable to a divorce rate. A true comparison would require looking at the total number and duration of relationships across a group of people's entire lifetimes, which, to my knowledge, has never been done.

Relationships are hard and all couples face conflicts about communication, intimacy, sex, finances, family issues, and household chores and responsibilities. Same-sex couples also face societal condemnation, possible lack of family support, and sometimes hostility from neighbors. These additional stresses can adversely affect a relationship. And as was noted earlier, internalized homophobia can affect the ability to form an intimate relationship. In Chapter 4, we will examine same-sex relationships in more detail, addressing such issues as the kinds of relationships that same-sex couples forge in the absence of marriage, the duration of relationships, and the factors that lead to breakup.

AREN'T HOMOSEXUALS OBSESSED WITH SEX?

Lesbian, gay, and bisexual people are usually defined by their sexuality: It is what sets them apart. Therefore, when homosexuality is mentioned, the first thing that most people think of is the sexual difference. Some people are fascinated or repelled by the idea of same-sex sexual acts. Research that has examined the frequency of sex or preferred sexual practices in heterosexual, gay, lesbian, and bisexual people shows more similarities than differences. And the few differences appear to fall along gender lines, rather than sexual identity lines. Men appear to think about, desire, and have sex more often than women. For example, Weinberg, Williams, and Pryor (1994) compared heterosexual, bisexual, and homosexual respondents from San Francisco sex organizations on a number of sexual behaviors and milestones. This is not a representative group and will overestimate the rates of some kinds of sexual experiences since these respondents were all contacted through organizations that cater to people with some kind of sexual interests. Also, the authors collected the data in San Francisco just at the beginning of the AIDS epidemic, before safer sex campaigns had really begun, and before we knew how HIV was transmitted. Nevertheless, the results are interesting and might represent trends in the general population as well. Table 3.1 shows some of the comparisons between heterosexuals, bisexuals, and homosexuals divided by gender.

The actual sexual practices that lesbian, gay, and bisexual people engage in are the same sexual practices that heterosexuals often enjoy—the only difference is the sex of the partner. There are no unique gay sex practices; lesbian, gay, and bisexual people often engage in kissing, caressing, manual stimulation of a partner's genitals, oral sex, vaginal sex, and anal intercourse. Sex plays the same role in the lives of lesbian, gay, and bisexual people as it does in the lives of heterosexuals. It can be the source of great pleasure and a means of deepening a relationship, but it can also cause pain and confusion.

LESBIAN, GAY, AND BISEXUAL PEOPLE "FLAUNT" THEIR SEXUALITY

A significant number of heterosexuals believe that lesbian, gay, and bisexual people are too "blatant" about their sexuality (see Chapter 2). Examples of flaunting include holding hands in public, putting a picture of a partner on the desk at work, bringing a partner to a work or family social event, wearing a t-shirt or button that proclaims sexual identity, or marching in a gay rights parade. Most heterosexuals fail to recognize that they can engage in these behaviors and more, and not be accused of "flaunting" their sexuality. Heterosexuals can flaunt their identities by putting their pictures in the newspaper to announce engagements, weddings, anniversaries, or divorces. They can safely put the picture of the spouse on their desk (in fact, it's almost expected of them) and hold hands anywhere. Heterosexuals often kiss goodbye in public places, and they even have heterosexual pride parades, such as the tradition of following the bride and groom's car around town after a wedding. Heterosexuals often wear wedding rings that publicly announce their sexual identity. Some people, regardless of their sexual identity, disregard notions of public decency and "make out" in public, but when heterosexuals accuse lesbian, gay, and bisexual

TABLE 3.1.　Comparison of Sexual Milestones and Sexual Practices in Heterosexuals, Bisexuals, and Homosexuals

MEN			
Sexual Milestone/Practice	Hetero (n=84)	Bisexual (n=116)	Gay (n=186)
Age of 1st heterosexual attraction	10.2	12.8	14.5 ($n = 52$)
Age of 1st heterosexual experience	16.7	15.9	17.7 ($n = 108$)
Age of 1st homosexual attraction	21.9 ($n = 25$)	17.1	11.5
Age of 1st homosexual experience	17.7 ($n = 40$)	17.2	14.7
Percent who ever felt confused about their sexuality	27	68	64
Median no. of sexual partners/past yr	2	4	6
Percent who performed oral sex/past yr	92	82	93
Percent who received oral sex/past yr	86	82	94
Percent who said lack of orgasm was a big problem	5	3-6	2

WOMEN			
Sexual Milestone/Practice	Hetero (n=104)	Bisexual (n=96)	Lesbian (n=94)
Age of 1st heterosexual attraction	10.4	10.9	14.3 ($n = 54$)
Age of 1st heterosexual experience	14.9	15.1	16.4 ($n = 73$)
Age of 1st homosexual attraction	23.6 ($n = 54$)	18.5	16.4
Age of 1st homosexual experience	23.0 ($n = 48$)	23.5	20.5
Percent who ever felt confused about their sexuality	28	76	67
Median no. of sexual partners/past yr	2	3	1
Percent who performed oral sex/past yr	93	75	89
Percent who received oral sex/past yr	89	74	90
Percent who said lack of orgasm was a big problem	15	9-11	7

Note. Adapted from Weinberg, Williams, and Pryor (1994).

people of flaunting, they are seldom referring to these offensive public sexual displays, but to behaviors that they can engage in without notice. Why are these same behaviors labeled as blatant flaunting when same-sex couples are involved?

HOMOSEXUALS COULD CHANGE THEIR PREFERENCE IF THEY TRIED

Silverstein (1991) noted that psychiatric diagnoses and treatments can be understood as a means of punishing people who violate social norms. Because of the tendency in modern society to label unconventional behavior as mental illness, psychiatric diagnoses change along with social norms and mores. For example, masturbation was considered an acceptable sexual behavior until doctors labeled it as a cause of insanity in the late 18th century. In the next century and a half, considerable efforts were made to "cure" masturbation, especially in children (John Kellogg's formula for corn flakes was supposed to inhibit sexual feelings in children). Society invents deviance, and psychiatric treatment and incarceration provide a means of controlling "deviants." When homosexuality was labeled as deviant in the late 1800s, psychiatry, religion, and the law all sought to contain it. The "cures" proposed by men of science included biological, medical, and psychological treatments that were based on a sickness model. Religious organizations, using the concept of sin, also offered conversion therapies based on prayer and development of strong moral character to overcome temptation.

T. F. Murphy (1992) reviewed some of the treatments aimed at redirecting sexual orientation. It appears that over the years, more efforts have been directed toward gay and bisexual men than toward lesbians or bisexual women, since men are traditionally more valued in our culture. Additionally, heterosexuality is defined by a certain kind of masculinity such that deviations from masculinity in men are more noticeable than deviations from femininity are in women, and more likely to be punished. Here are some of the treatments that Murphy discovered for redirecting male homosexuality:

- Excessive bicycle riding (to make the patient too tired to think about sex).

- Rest from the stresses of urban living.
- Visits to prostitutes.
- Marriage and/or sex with "virtuous" women.
- Masturbating to pictures of women.
- Sensate focus (Masters and Johnson's therapy, which included a gradual progression of eye contact, communication, relaxation, body exploration, and eventually vaginal intercourse).
- Home versions of electroshock programs.
- Threat of beatings.
- The mental equivalent of excessive physical exercise (intensive academic study designed to exhaust the patient).
- Psychoanalysis of a variety of sorts (overcoming fear of women, overcoming dependency on mother, resolving early childhood conflicts, etc.).
- Bible study and religious conversion.
- X-ray treatments.
- Hydrotherapy.
- Acupuncture.
- Hypnosis.
- Assertiveness training.
- Primal screaming.
- Training in the "beauty" of the opposite sex.
- Exorcism.
- Drug therapy of a variety of sorts.
- Surgeries (castration, testicle transplants, lobotomy, cauterization of neck, lower back, and groin, destruction of diencephalon).

Murphy also reported that in the late 1800s a physician who believed that lesbianism was a class phenomenon—an affliction of the "idle rich" not found in the working classes—treated lesbianism with a cocaine solution combined with a "saline cathartic," "bromides, sometimes combined with cannabis indica," or an injection of strychnine. Other treatments for lesbianism have included clitoral amputation and many of the other treatments noted for gay men.

Hormonal drug treatments, such as testosterone injections for gay men (which did not initiate desire for women, but increased the desire for men) and estrogen treatment for lesbians were based on the idea that deficient sex hormones were responsible for causing homosexuality, despite the lack of evidence for hormonal differences. Psychological treatments have included psychoanalysis to resolve conflicts of early childhood thought to underlie homosexuality; conditioning treatments, as in aversion therapies where unpleasant stimuli such as shocks are given when the client has a sexual response to someone of the same sex; and cognitive therapies that emphasize the powers of the mind over the body (you can be heterosexual if you just try hard enough).

Murphy noted that nearly every study that has reported success in redirecting sexual orientation has been seriously flawed (e.g., not including a control group, having only short-term follow-up, or not adequately defining the sexuality of the clients). Most sound studies suggest that no treatment is effective for changing sexual orientation, although specific sexual behaviors can be modified at least on a short-term basis.

DIDN'T HOMOSEXUALS BRING AIDS TO THE UNITED STATES?

Since the start of the AIDS epidemic in the United States, lesbian, gay, and bisexual people (especially gay and bisexual men) have been accused of bringing this terminal illness to the general population. Unlike other countries of the world, where AIDS is primarily transmitted by heterosexual sex, in the United States the first wave of transmission disproportionately affected gay and bisexual men. AIDS is a sexually transmitted disease and it took a few years to spread into the heterosexual population in the United States (Stine, 1995). Because of this early history, stereotypes about AIDS involve gay people and include:

- All lesbian, gay, and bisexual people have AIDS (assuming that sexual identity is the "risk factor").
- Gay men are responsible for bringing AIDS to the United States.
- AIDS is God's punishment for homosexuality.
- People with deviant sexual practices have to suffer the consequences of their acts (they get what they deserve).
- No money should be given to AIDS research, because if gay men stopped having sex, there would be no more AIDS.

Such stereotypes are unfounded. They assume that HIV has a moral connotation, however, viruses can affect anyone. If AIDS hadn't started in the gay and bisexual men's communities, it would have started somewhere else, perhaps in predominantly heterosexual communities as it did in Africa. If AIDS is God's punishment for homosexuality, then He is very selective, as lesbians continue to have very low rates of HIV infection (they are not immune to AIDS by any means, but their rates of HIV are much lower than in gay or bisexual men). The idea that people get what they deserve would need to be extended to other risky behaviors. For example, perhaps no money should be given for lung cancer research, because smokers get what they deserve, or no resources should be extended to people with colon cancers who ate too much fat in their diets. Perhaps liver transplants should not be offered to people like Mickey Mantle or Larry Hagman who "purposely" damaged their livers via alcohol abuse.

These AIDS stereotypes manifest in health care providers who take extraordinary precautions when they know their patient is lesbian, gay, or bisexual. Universal precautions must be used with every patient, but using special care with selected patients is insulting and humiliating to them. In the summer of 1995, a group of elected lesbian, gay, and bisexual representatives and senators were invited to the White House for a meeting. When they arrived, they were greeted by Secret Service members wearing rubber gloves. None of these people were known to have AIDS, and even if they had been, they were unlikely to have engaged in any risky behaviors during their White House visit. AIDS hysteria still exists, despite our knowing for many years now that HIV cannot be transmitted via casual contact. AIDS will be discussed in more detail in Chapter 8.

AREN'T BISEXUALS JUST CONFUSED ABOUT THEIR IDENTITIES?

Most of the previously discussed stereotypes also apply to bisexuals, but some additional myths are specific to bisexuality:

• Bisexuals are confused or are fence-sitters.
• Bisexuals are gay or lesbian people who are afraid to admit it.

- Bisexuals want the best of both worlds.
- Bisexuals brought AIDS into heterosexual and lesbian communities.
- Bisexuals must always have a partner of each sex at one time.
- Bisexuals cannot commit—they will always leave you for someone of the other sex.
- Bisexuals are "trendy"—it's just a fad or a phase.

Many of these myths come from our simplistic binary system; things are black or white, right or wrong, male or female, and heterosexual or homosexual. Bisexuals do not fit into this equation (nor do people of intermediate skin tones or mixed racial heritage). The binary system denies the legitimacy of a bisexual identity and assumes that people have to choose heterosexuality or homosexuality. As bisexuality moves into the mainstream, people are forced to consider the fluidity of sexuality (Garber, 1995).

Weinberg, Williams, and Pryor's (1994) study of bisexuals in San Francisco revealed that bisexuals are no more often confused about their sexuality than lesbian or gay people (and even a substantial number of heterosexuals had been confused about their sexuality at some time). They also found that bisexuals were more like lesbian, gay, and heterosexual people than unlike. Most bisexuals experienced serial monogamy (one sexual partner at a time), and most bisexuals experienced their sexual identity as relatively stable (they identified as bisexual, not as undecided).

Biphobia, or negative attitudes about bisexual people, differs somewhat from homophobia, although they are closely related forms of prejudice. A small, but significant number of gay and lesbian people are biphobic, although few are overtly homophobic. Some lesbian and gay people are biphobic as a result of their own internalized homophobia, which causes them to lash out at others who are "different." Others are suspicious of bisexuals because they have internalized the stereotypes about bisexuals being unstable, untrustworthy, and as "closeted" lesbians and gay men. Some lesbian feminists consider bisexual women as traitors—they are "sleeping with the enemy." In a recent study (Eliason, 1996c), 30% of heterosexual respondents were biphobic compared with 5% of lesbian and gay respondents.

CONCLUSION

In this chapter, I have discussed several common stereotypes about lesbian, gay, and bisexual people. Stereotypes are fragmented, usually inaccurate, pieces of information about some group of people based on an assumption that everyone in the group is alike or interchangeable. Stereotypes deny group members their humanity and uniqueness. Most stereotypes about lesbian, gay, and bisexual people are negative, and have obvious adverse effects. Even positive stereotypes, however, can have adverse effects. If a stereotype about gay men is that they are all good-looking and sensitive, what happens to the gay man who does not fit into our norms of physical attractiveness or is just average in sensitivity? Might he feel inadequate? If stereotypes about bisexual people state that they are more sexually experienced and promiscuous than other people, can the bisexual woman who has not yet had sex with either a man or a woman identify herself as bisexual?

Breaking down stereotypical thinking is difficult, because we seem to seek the easiest possible solutions. Thinking in terms of stereotypes is simple, whereas considering each person as a unique being and taking the time and energy to get to know that person is exhausting, although potentially rewarding.

EXERCISE: EXPLORING STEREOTYPES

Think about the stereotypes you learned about lesbian, gay, or bisexual people when you were growing up. For example, can you remember the first time you realized that there were lesbian, gay, or bisexual people in the world? Think about that incident and remember what kind of feelings you had about it at the time. What did your family, teachers, or friends say about lesbian, gay, or bisexual people? Was anyone at your school labeled as "queer?" If so, how was that person treated? Did children in your school use terms like "fag" or "fairy?" What effects did these names have on you?

Imagine that tomorrow at work, a co-worker says something that indicates a sexual identity stereotype, such as commenting that gay men are child molesters. What do you think you would do or say?

CHAPTER FOUR

Lesbian, Gay, and Bisexual Family Issues

IN 1993, SHARON BOTTOMS, A 23-year-old mother of a two-year-old son, lost custody of her child. According to court testimony, she was a good mother to Tyler and provided a stable home. So why did she lose her child? The first judge to hear the case ruled that because she was in a relationship with a woman, and in her home state of Virginia, lesbian sexual relationships are against the law, that Sharon Bottoms was a criminal and thus could not be a good mother. Although the Court of Appeals overturned that ruling in favor of Sharon, in 1995, the Virginia Supreme Court ruled that the separation was in the best interests of the child; not because Sharon was a bad mother, but because Tyler might face social stigma because of his mother's "lifestyle." Ironically, Sharon testified that she herself was sexually abused in her mother's home by her mother's live-in boyfriend, the same environment her son is now experiencing.

This story is all too common among lesbian, gay, and bisexual people. Although "society" often is hostile to lesbian, gay, and bisexual people, in this case, Sharon Bottom's own mother filed suit against her and took her child. Some same-sex families face rejection, harassment, discrimination, and even violence from within their families of origin. As lesbian, gay, and bisexual families become more visible in society, and as research continues to show that same-sex couples can and usually do provide good homes for their children, loss of custody based solely on sexual orientation is becoming somewhat less common. Custody battles, however, are only one highly visible assault on lesbian, gay, and bisexual families.

Same-sex couples do not have the rights afforded to married heterosexual couples: they cannot sue a third party for wrongful death of a
partner, they cannot qualify for family insurance plans, and they do
not qualify for exemption from probate that is offered to married
spouses. Persons who are known to be lesbian, gay, or bisexual cannot
immigrate or bring a foreign partner to the United States nor can they
apply for citizenship for their partners. Some areas have zoning laws
that restrict the number of unrelated persons living in "single-family
dwellings." Military regulations mean that same-sex partners cannot be
stationed together: To reveal their relationship would mean probable
discharge from the service (Weston, 1991).

Health care providers need to be aware of these realities. In this
chapter, I will present current knowledge about lesbian, gay, and bisexual families, and suggest ways that health care providers can work
effectively with them. It is likely that most health care providers *have*
worked with lesbian, gay, or bisexual families, whether or not they are
aware of it. It is difficult to identify the actual number of lesbian, gay,
or bisexual family units in the population for many reasons, some of
which were touched on in Chapter 1. Common societal definitions of
family may exclude same-sex couples. For example, if family is defined
by blood relationships or legal marriage ties, lesbian, gay, and bisexual
families will not be counted. If family is defined as having at least one
child, same-sex childless couples are excluded. Even when family is defined more broadly, such as two or more people who provide emotional and/or financial support for each other, lesbian, gay, and
bisexual relationships have been rendered virtually invisible because
of negative societal attitudes and the potential for discrimination. If a
bisexual person is in a relationship with a person of the other sex, that
relationship appears to be heterosexual, carries all the privileges of
heterosexuality, but renders the bisexuality of one or both partners invisible. When a bisexual person is in a relationship with someone of
the same sex, the relationship is treated as a gay or lesbian union, again
erasing the bisexuality of one or both partners.

One reason for the silence of some same-sex couples is the risk of
loss of family. Court custody cases are still rarely won by lesbian, gay,
or bisexual parents (Falk, 1989), and adoption agencies and foster care
institutions still hesitate to allow same-sex couples to raise children
(Ricketts & Achtenberg, 1990). When a same-sex couple coparents a

child born to one of them, the nonbiological parent seldom wins the right to adopt the child (Burke, 1993).

Estimates of the number of lesbian, gay, and bisexual people and families are difficult to obtain because sexual orientation is not a visible marker like gender or race. Many lesbian and gay people choose not to reveal their sexual orientation to health care workers, teachers, or others who might have a negative impact on their lives. Until it is safe to come out in public, there will be no accurate estimates of the number of lesbian, gay, and bisexual people in the country.

Keeping these limitations in mind, several recent studies have estimated that the number of same-sex couples with children includes 1 to 5 million lesbian mothers (Falk, 1989; Gottman, 1990; Pennington, 1987) and 1 to 3 million gay male parents (Bozett, 1987; Gottman, 1990). These parenthood rates could mean that 6 to 14 million children are currently being raised in same-sex households (Editors, *Harvard Law Review,* 1990). These estimates, which are based on the number of lesbian and gay people who have children from previous heterosexual marriages, may be an underestimate because they do not include children from the "lesbian baby boom" (lesbians who have babies after "coming out" as lesbians), or children who come from adoption, foster care, and coparenting (Alpert, 1988; McCandlish, 1987; Pies, 1985; Pollach & Vaughn, 1987). Patterson (1994) has suggested that there may be as many as 8 million gay and lesbian parents in the United States, and many more childless lesbian and gay couple families.

FAMILY OF ORIGIN ISSUES

The majority of lesbian, gay, and bisexual people are raised in heterosexual households with parents whose dreams for their children include heterosexual marriage and parenthood. Thus, disclosure to family is a major stressor in the coming out process. Families are a major source of support for most people, so concerns about familial rejection or disappointing one's parents are prevalent and intense.

For parents of a lesbian, gay, or bisexual child, the coming out process can include an initial feeling of guilt or sense of failure as a parent (Griffin, Wirth, & Wirth, 1986). This feeling of having done something wrong can stem in part from psychoanalytic theories that blame parents for their children's homosexuality by stating that mothers have been too overprotective, or too distant, or treated their children in gender-inappropriate ways, or that fathers have been too distant or failed to appropriately socialize their children. Although none of these psychoanalytic theories have been proven to be true, they can influence our thinking about homosexuality and wrongly place the burden of guilt on parents.

The guilt phase is often followed by stereotypical thinking, in which parents apply negative stereotypes about lesbian, gay, and bisexual people to their own child (thus thinking of that child as a stranger). Their fear of rejection, ridicule, or disapproval from other family members, friends, members of the church, or the community can lead to isolation and social withdrawal. A child's coming out of the closet may ironically push parents and other family members into one. The lesbian, gay, or bisexual child has probably had several months or years to come to terms with her/his own sexuality, but other family members may be quite unprepared for the disclosure.

The third stage of the process can include feeling alienated from the lesbian, gay, or bisexual child, and perhaps resentful about the disruption of family relationships. Finally, some parents resolve their conflicts by rejecting the negative stereotypes and accepting that their child is still the same one they have loved for years.

One parent described her daughter's coming out as follows:

I had known a few homosexuals along life's way and I was not aware of feeling any prejudice against them. I was comfortable in their presence, and we got along well. In fact, when one of our good friends came to us and told us he was gay, we found that our relationship was strengthened rather than weakened.

Then, when my daughter Robin was about twenty-one, she told me she was gay. It hit me like the proverbial ton of bricks. I was devastated. How could I have brought such a thing on my child? Where had I gone wrong? I immediately assumed responsibility for her gayness.

I was quite surprised by my reactions; I would not have thought I would take it so hard. After all, I was an "enlightened woman." I even had a close friend who. . . . I realized then that we can't predict how we will react to a given situation, even though we may think ourselves capable of handling it. How much harder it is to deal with information when it hits us emotionally than when we view it intellectually! So I hadn't really escaped my conditioning; I had merely covered it over. It was still deep within me, ready to surface when I got "hit" emotionally. . . . It took a while to readjust my thinking, to gain perspective, and finally, to ask myself what I really wanted for my daughter. When I realized that I really wanted her to find happiness, love, and fulfillment in her own way, I found that I was "OK," and I felt that I had "arrived." (Fairchild & Hayward, 1989, pp. 48–49)

Not all parents respond with loving support of their children. Recent data suggest that between 25% and 40% of runaway teens are lesbian, gay, or bisexual and have been rejected by their families, or feared violence from their families if they disclosed (Due, 1995). Hunter (1994) found that 61% of gay-related violence against teenagers came from their own families.

A survey of over 100 lesbians with an average age of 37 found that 24% reported that parental acceptance of their lesbianism was a major problem and 47% said it was some problem (Eliason & Morgan, 1996b). Parental acceptance is an issue not only for adolescents or young adults—some lesbian, gay, and bisexual people feel pressured to keep the secret from their parents or grandparents most of their lives. To keep the secret, however, children must shut out a significant part of their lives from parents or other family members. Other families live with an "open secret"—they know about the homosexuality or bisexuality but refuse to discuss it openly. These family situations create many awkward situations for coupled lesbian, gay, and bisexual people who may need to introduce significant others as friends or roommates. This charade with family can seriously strain the relationship.

There is very little empirical research about the reactions of parents, the means by which they resolve conflict and achieve understanding, or how long the process of acceptance takes. In larger cities, there are organizations for parents such as PFLAG (Parents and Friends of Lesbians and Gays) that offer education and support and can speed the process. Most families, however, face these issues alone. There is little research on the reactions of siblings, grandparents, best friends, or other people close to the disclosing lesbian, gay, or bisexual person. Jones (1978) suggested that siblings react much like their parents except for not feeling guilt or self-blame. Lesbian, gay, and bisexual people often disclose to a trusted sibling before coming out to parents (Strommen, 1989).

Fairchild and Hayward (1989) provided many suggestions to parents of children who have just come out. Some of the suggestions could apply equally well to health care providers and their clients/patients:

- Talk to others about it; don't keep this a dark family secret.
- Relax—it's not the end of the world, just another life transition.
- Reassure your child—she/he is probably afraid of your possible rejection.
- Continue to enjoy your child as a unique human being—she/he is not different, just more honest.
- Support your child in her/his decisions.
- Be patient—it takes time to adjust.
- Don't suggest a "cure"—it sends the message that you think the child is sick.
- Don't suggest it's a fad or phase—your child probably thought about it for a very long time before telling you, so don't trivialize it.
- Get informed—read, talk to others, find out as much as you can.

A significant number of lesbian, gay, and bisexual people enter heterosexual marriages before coming out (about 20% of gay men and 33% of lesbians). Reasons for marriage include the belief that homosexual feelings were just a phase, a lack of awareness of homosexual feelings at the time of the marriage, a belief that marriage would "cure" homosexuality, desire for children, and genuine love for the spouse (Strommen, 1989). Some lesbian and gay people decide not to come out and must lead double lives, whereas others feel the need to be honest with their spouse. The reactions of the heterosexual spouse are extremely varied, but coming out often leads to divorce (Bozett, 1982; Coleman, 1985a, 1985b). Occasionally, however, the disclosure leads to greater intimacy and closeness in the relationship, and it evolves into an open marriage or an asexual partnership (Brownfain, 1985; Gochros, 1989). Bisexual women and men are more likely to remain in a marriage after coming out than are lesbian or gay individuals (Brownfain, 1985). Strommen (1989) suggested that gay men come out to wives or exwives more often than lesbians come out to husbands because husbands or exhusbands are more likely to respond with anger and/or violence, and lesbians fear loss of custody of children more.

GAY AND LESBIAN COUPLES AS CHOSEN FAMILY

There is little evidence that same-sex couples are fundamentally different from other-sex couples in any way except for the treatment they receive from society (Peplau, 1993). Kurdek (1994) found that 40%–60% of gay men and 45%–80% of lesbians are in long-term, stable relationships, and he found that relationship satisfaction was similar to that found in heterosexual couples (see also Duffy & Rusbult, 1985/1986). Although same-sex relationships are at high risk for conflict and dissolution, nearly half of heterosexual marriages end in divorce. This is not a fair comparison, however, because heterosexual marriage and divorce rates do not reflect the number of failed relationships a heterosexual person might have had before marriage. Although same-sex couples do not have the legal marker of a marriage by which to judge their relationships, they provide largely the same reasons for failure as other-sex couples, including conflicts about finances, communication problems, infidelity, and growing apart. In addition, the same-sex couple has the burden of societal disapproval and lack of privileges that accompany legal marriages, such as tax benefits, health insurance coverage, and inheritance. The partners may be at different stages of coming out, have conflicting attitudes about how open they should be as a couple, and experience differing levels of internalized homophobia.

Social Support for Same-Sex Couples

Same-sex couples may also have different forms of social support than heterosexual couples. For example, Aura (1985) found that heterosexual women relied heavily on relatives for support, whereas lesbians were more likely to turn to partners and friends. Kurdek (1988), however, found that gay men and lesbians often cited family members as a major source of support, showing that family support is certainly present for many same-sex couples, though not to the same extent as for heterosexual couples. Lesbians may also rely on feminist organizations and peers for social support (Leavy & Adams, 1986). This latter study also found that being in a relationship was positively associated with social support and higher self-esteem in lesbians.

When social support is lacking from families of origin, lesbian, gay, and bisexual people forge closer, more familial ties with friends and lovers. Nardi and Sherrod (1994) surveyed 161 gay men and 122 lesbians from Los Angeles (mostly white, well-educated, and around the age of 40). As a group, they placed high value on their friendships; gay men and lesbians spent about equal amounts of time with their friends, had similar levels of satisfaction with their friendships, and were equally disclosing and emotionally expressive with their friends. Among the few differences by gender, lesbians reported being more bothered by conflicts with friends and resolved conflict by expressing how they felt about it. Gay men were less bothered by conflict and resolved it by talking about the situation or ignoring it. Another difference was in the likelihood of having sex with a friend. Gay men were more likely to have sex with casual or close friends, but not best friends. Lesbians were twice as likely to report that their current lover was their best friend. When lesbian, gay, or bisexual people are hospitalized, friends may serve the same support function that family members serve for hospitalized heterosexual people. Health care providers need to recognize the value of close friends in the recovery process.

Same-Sex Couple Relationship Characteristics

Bryant and Demian (1994) reported on one of the largest surveys of same-sex couples to date. This national study included 560 male couples (97% gay and 3% bisexual partners) and 706 female couples (93% lesbian and 7% bisexual partners). Men reported longer current relationships than did women (an average of 7 years for the men compared with 5 years for the women), and 25% of the men had been in the same relationship for more than 10 years, compared with 14% of the women. The majority of couples reported being committed to making their current relationship long-term (92% of the women and 96% of the men). Women were more likely to have had some type of commitment ceremony or ritual, and to wear a ring or other symbol of the relationship than were men. Women also rated the quality of their relationships higher than men.

Bryant and Demian asked about the terms the couples preferred to use for their significant others. Women preferred "partner" or "life partner" (37%) and men preferred "lover" (40%). A significant number had previously been involved in heterosexual marriages (27% of the women; 19% of the men), and many had already had three or more previous serious relationships (19% of the women; 11% of the men).

More of the women reported sexually exclusive relationships (90%) than men (63%), and although men reported having sex more frequently (on average, 10 times per month), women reported enjoying sex with their partner more (and had sex on average, 7 times per month). In fact, 54% of the women and 34% of the men rated the quality of sex in their relationships as excellent, although satisfaction with sex tended to decrease with relationship length. Only 2% of the women, compared with 22% of the men reported having sex outside the relationship.

Women and men tended to meet their partners in different places. Women met their current partners through friends (28%) or at work (21%), but not often at bars (4%) or other sexually charged arenas such as bathhouses or through classified ads (9%). Men met their partners in those sexually charged arenas (39%), bars (22%), through friends (19%), and rarely, at work (7%). Bryant and Demian reported that men and women faced the same main challenges to the relationships. Both sexes cited communication problems as the major problem, followed by conflicts about career, relatives, sex, and finances.

Relationship Satisfaction and Sources of Conflict

Several studies have found that relationship satisfaction is generally high and does not differ for female and male same-sex couples on global measures of satisfaction (Duffy & Rusbult, 1985/1986). However, if the measure is of the perceived value of the relationship and the rewards derived from it, female same-sex couples generally report higher relationship satisfaction than males (Blumstein & Schwartz, 1983). Kurdek (1995) suggested that this finding is consistent with women's greater socialization to value relationships. In support of this, Kurdek found that gay men are more like heterosexual married men in their ratings of relationship satisfaction whereas lesbians are more like heterosexual married women. Additionally, the factors that predict relationship satisfaction tend to be similar for all types of couples (male and female same-sex couples and married and unmarried other-sex couples): a perception of equality in power and control in the relationship,

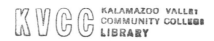

having at least one partner who is emotionally expressive, sharing in decision making, satisfaction with levels of affection and sex, high levels of commitment to the relationship, relatively few conflicts, financial security and legal preparedness, and placing value on the relationship (Bryant & Demian, 1994; Kurdek, 1995). Same-sex couples are likely to share household responsibilities equally or divide tasks according to partner preferences or skills rather than along gender role lines.

Some authors have proposed that there are predictable stages in a couple relationship. Table 4.1 depicts the model proposed by McWhirter and Mattison (1984) which was originally based on data from gay male couples. Kurdek and Schmitt (1986) successfully applied the model to female and male same-sex couples and other-sex couples, finding that couples in the nesting phase reported the lowest satisfaction with the relationship, the greatest stress, and the most disillusionment. There were no differences between same-sex and other-sex couples in the stages of their relationships.

Sexual exclusivity in the relationship is an area of major difference between male and female same-sex couples. Male couples are more likely to tolerate, have, and sometimes value, extrarelationship sex (Bryant & Demian, 1994; Kurdek, 1995), although rates of sexual exclusivity appear to have increased in men since the rise of the AIDS epidemic (Kurdek, 1995).

TABLE 4.1.   Stages in Same-Sex Couple Relationships

Years	Phase	Description
1	Blending	Merging, shared activities, high sexual activity
2–3	Nesting	Homemaking, finding compatibility, ambivalence about the relationship
4–5	Maintaining	Learning to deal with conflict, establishing traditions, re-emergence of the individual
6–10	Building	Collaborating, establishing independence, acknowledging dependability of partners
11–20	Releasing	Trusting each other, merging money and possessions, taking each other for granted
20+	Renewing	Financial and emotional security, restoring romance

Note. Adapted from McWhirter and Mattison (1984).

Relationship conflicts seem to stem from the same sources in same- and other-sex couples, and include finances, driving style, expression of affection and sex, being overly critical, and division of labor of household tasks (Kurdek, 1995). When a relationship dissolves, it is often because of nonresponsiveness of one partner or increased emotional distance. Same-sex partners react to a breakup with the same emotional responses as other-sex partners—loneliness, relief from conflict, financial stress, and feeling personal growth.

The unique problem of internalized homophobia may put lesbian and gay couples at risk by causing one or both partners to experience distrust, loneliness, difficulty establishing and maintaining intimate relationships, under- or overachievement, impaired sexual functioning, domestic violence, poor coping, unsafe sexual experiences, alcohol and drug abuse, depression, and suicide. These negative consequences can put a tremendous strain on the relationship. Self-hatred and a positive, intimate relationship are usually incompatible, yet in some cases, the strength of love and support from a partner may help the individual to overcome internalized homophobia. Focusing the blame on negative societal attitudes rather than the person's own shortcomings or a partner's faults can strengthen the relationship.

Other health care issues faced by lesbian and gay couples include when or whether to disclose their sexual orientation to a health care provider, stresses that arise when one partner is ill or injured, violence within and outside the relationship, the risk for hospitalization for gay-bashing episodes, care of a partner with AIDS, and hospital policies or procedures that may discriminate against same-sex partners.

Disclosure of Sexual Identity to Health Care Providers

Next to disclosure of sexual identity to parents, disclosure to a health care provider can be one of the most stressful events in a lesbian, gay, or bisexual person's life. This is a difficult and complex issue because while it is important to give health care providers complete, honest, and accurate information, such providers can have negative attitudes that may compromise health care delivery. In some cases, the lesbian, gay, or bisexual person can choose to disclose or not, but in emergency situations, the disclosure may be involuntary or unavoidable. In 1983, when Sharon Kowalski was seriously injured in a car accident, her life partner, Karen Thompson, was unable to obtain any information on her partner's condition until Sharon's parents arrived because she was not a blood relative or a legal spouse. Finally, she revealed their relationship, not knowing whether Sharon would approve, but hoping that health care providers and Sharon's family would better understand her need to be involved in Sharon's recovery. Instead, Sharon's family reacted with denial and legally prevented Karen from visiting Sharon (for more details, see Thompson and Andrzejewski, 1988, and Chapter 1 of this book). Although disclosure may be necessary for participation in the health care of a partner, Sharon and Karen's story shows how it can generate serious problems and put the same-sex couple at risk for harassment and discrimination.

Many lesbian, gay, and bisexual people worry that health care providers will not take their relationships as seriously as heterosexual relationships. One lesbian wrote:

> *Psychosocial health care issues are of concern to me, e.g., although my partner and I have durable power of attorney papers in our medical records, I worry that even if the letter of the law is honored, that the spirit of the law won't be honored. Health care providers still don't get that we're not pals, buddies, roommates, girlfriends, or old maids, etc. I don't believe that in the case of serious illness, death, or serious treatment decisions that they comprehend we share the fears that any spouse would have. I haven't found the same compassion offered to me when my partner was hospitalized as was extended to heterosexual spouses. (Eliason & Morgan, 1996c, p. 11)*

Partners may disagree about the need for disclosure, adding another source of stress to the illness or to their relationship. Because of the issue's importance, I will discuss disclosure to health care providers in detail in Chapter 5.

Violence and Same-Sex Couples

Violence based on sexual identity prejudice is a unique problem for lesbian, gay, and bisexual people. Violence against lesbian, gay, and bisexual people is not new: laws in 13th-century Europe punished sodomy with castration and/or death; Nazi party members incarcerated and murdered between 5,000 and 15,000 lesbian and gay people in concentration camps; police have brutalized and raped lesbian, gay, and bisexual people who were arrested only for congregating in gay bars (Herek & Berrill, 1992). Virtually all openly lesbian, gay, or bisexual people have experienced some form of victimization, such as verbal abuse, threats, being chased or followed, or being spat on. Gay-bashing is physical violence directed at a person solely on the basis of the individual's perceived sexual orientation, and affects about 20% of lesbian, gay, and bisexual people in their lifetimes (Herek & Birrell, 1992). As if the physical violence were not traumatic enough, many suffer secondary victimization from police and health care workers who question what the injured person did to "deserve" the violence (a form of victim blaming), or do not believe that the violence was gay-bashing, but characterize it as a random act of violence (Cotton, 1992).

The victim of hate violence and her/his partner may need extra support services to deal with its consequences. According to Garnets, Herek, and Levy (1990), the psychological aftermath of antigay violence can include sleep disturbances, nightmares, diarrhea, headaches, relationship problems, increased drug use, and decreased levels of trust and safety. Some people react to violence with self-blame and feelings of worthlessness. Others question why it happened to them—what did I do wrong? Severely afflicted individuals may develop Post-traumatic Stress Disorder, a syndrome defined by persistent reexperiencing of the trauma, persistent avoidance of trauma-associated stimuli, numbing of general emotional expression, and persistent symptoms of stress. The symptoms may abate over time, but the time to recover is highly variable. High levels of internalized homophobia may aggravate the symptoms. If sexual assault occurred, the consequent feelings of humiliation and degradation may affect current or future sexual relationships. Garnets et al. (1990) provided some suggestions for health care providers dealing with victims of antigay violence:

- Respect confidentiality.
- Assure physical safety of the victim.
- Assess coping skills and social support.
- Know referral sources in the gay community.
- Listen, and don't question why it happened.

- Allow victims to express anger toward the assailant.
- Link the violence to homophobia (help decrease self-blame).
- Incorporate significant others into the healing process.

Domestic violence potentially affects all types of relationships. About 25%–33% of people in heterosexual relationships report at least one incident of domestic violence to the authorities, and estimates of the actual occurrence of violence in intimate relationships is much higher than the reported cases (Koss, 1990). Since men are more likely to perpetrate violence and, overall, violence between men is more common than male-female violence, it is not surprising that domestic violence may be a significant problem in male same-sex couples. Ireland and Letellier (1991) suggested that some degree of violence may occur in nearly 50% of male-male couples. For the same reasons, lesbian couples may have lower rates of violence than gay male or heterosexual couples, although lesbians are not immune to domestic violence by any means. The increased levels of stress and lack of relationship role norms may place lesbians at about the same risk of battering as heterosexual women (Renzetti, 1992). When domestic violence does occur, lesbian, gay, and bisexual victims may not know where to go for help because most domestic violence shelters are geared toward heterosexual women. Because shelter workers assume that men are batterers, they are confused by lesbian victims of battering, and are likely to put the blame on the battered lesbian herself (Renzetti, 1992). Other shelter workers or shelter residents may be homophobic, creating a hostile environment for lesbian battering victims. Few resources are available at all for battered gay or bisexual men.

Living with Illness or Disability

When one partner has HIV or AIDS, the family involved will need considerable support. AIDS care is beyond the scope of this chapter, but I will cover it in more detail in Chapter 8. Many lesbian, gay, and bisexual people fear that health care providers who do not take their relationships seriously will not offer adequate support to a grieving partner. Illness or disability in a partner can trigger significant emotional responses that impair the partner's ability to cope and may create problems for the staff.

Hospitalization

When a partner in a same-sex relationship must be hospitalized, many hospitals still have policies that exclude the partner from visiting or receiving information. Some emergency rooms and intensive care units only allow blood relatives or legal spouses to visit. Even when partners are allowed access to the ill or injured party, they are not guaranteed the same respect given to legal spouses. Partners may be ignored, avoided, or disparaged. Hospital admission forms may not have spaces to designate partners or to acknowledge legal documents such as durable power of attorney for health care. Health care providers need to recognize the value of significant others in the recovery process and redefine these policies—does it really matter if the person is a blood relative or legal spouse? Isn't the point to have a familiar and caring person to support the ill one? I will discuss these issues in Chapter 9.

There are some signs that our society is beginning to change and to value committed families of many forms. Some companies, universities, and cities are beginning to recognize the value of relationships for same-sex couples by providing domestic partner benefits or beginning registries for domestic partners. These policies validate the seriousness of lesbian and gay unions by putting them on a near-equal basis with marriage. In an era when "family values" are touted as the solution for societal problems, loving, committed relationships of all kinds need to be valued and encouraged. Savvy business owners know that employee satisfaction is partially based on the benefits of the employment and that offering domestic partner benefits costs them very little but improves employee morale, which in turn, improves productivity.

LESBIAN, GAY, AND BISEXUAL FAMILIES WITH CHILDREN

Issues That May Affect Children

Objections to same-sex couples raising children range from stereotypes about child molestation or emotional instability to the belief that children must have mother and father role models for complete, normal development. Another fear is that the children will grow up to be lesbian, gay, or bisexual themselves. Even among people who accept adult lesbian and gay relationships, a significant number object to lesbian, gay, or bisexual people raising children. They state that adults can choose to lead stigmatized lives, but that children should be protected from undue hardship (this was the argument the Virginia Supreme Court used in deciding the Sharon Bottoms' case cited earlier). Others might argue that divorce, child abuse, and parental alcoholism and drug abuse are also undue hardships, but although these problems occur at a high rate in heterosexual families, no one blames these problems on heterosexuality per se. Is there a basis for the common belief that children of lesbian, gay, or bisexual parents suffer more hardship or develop differently than children of heterosexual parents?

Although research on lesbian, gay, and bisexual family units is relatively recent, the results of the studies have been fairly consistent: The vast majority of studies find no differences between children raised by lesbian, gay, or bisexual parents and children raised by heterosexual parents. The following paragraphs briefly summarize these findings.

Gender Identity. There are no differences in children's sense of themselves as female or male if they are raised by lesbian or gay parents or heterosexual parents (Golombok, Spencer, & Rutter, 1983; Kirkpatrick, Smith, & Roy, 1981).

Gender Role Behavior. Defined as gender stereotypical toy choice, preferred activities, and interests, most studies indicate no gender role differences between children of lesbian and gay parents and children of heterosexuals (Green, 1978; Gottman, 1990; Hoeffer, 1981). One study however (Green, Mandel, Hotvedt, Gray, & Smith, 1986), found that children of lesbian mothers were less rigidly gender typed in their activities and had a wider range of interests. This may be a major advantage of same-sex families—their children may be freer to explore their own unique personalities with less adherence to gender role stereotypes. The child whose two fathers share all household responsibilities may learn a valuable lesson about cooperation and equality in a relationship. The child whose two mothers both work outside the home and share lawn-mowing as well as cooking may learn to value women's contributions to society more. Children of lesbian, gay, and bisexual parents may be more likely to learn that your gender does not restrict who and what you can be in this world—that men can be sensitive and that women can be assertive.

Sexual Orientation.   None of several studies have found a higher incidence of homosexuality, or signs thought to predict homosexuality, in
children raised by lesbian or gay parents (Golombok, Spencer, & Rutter, 1983; Huggins, 1989). A few studies have examined adult children
of gay and lesbian parents with the same results—they have found the
base rate of homosexuality in the general population (8%–16%)
(Gottman, 1990; Miller, 1979; Paul, 1986). These findings are rather
surprising in light of numerous studies that propose a genetic basis for
homosexuality. If that were true, you would expect to see a higher rate
of homosexuality and bisexuality in the children of lesbian, gay, and bisexual parents. Another factor that contributes to the notion that parents have little influence on their children's sexual identity is that
most lesbian, gay, and bisexual people have been raised by heterosexual parents. There is strong evidence that parenting does not influence
sexual identity formation.

Personality Development.   Most studies find no difference in rates of
psychiatric or behavioral problems, self-esteem, or other personality
measures (Golombok, Spencer, & Rutter, 1983; Gottman, 1990; Huggins, 1989). However, in one small-scale study of 11 preschool children of lesbian mothers compared with 11 preschool children of
heterosexual couples, the children of heterosexual parents were rated
as more aggressive, bossy, domineering, and negative. The children of
lesbian mothers were rated as more lovable, affectionate, responsive
and protective toward younger children (Steckel, 1985, 1987). The results of this very small study must be viewed with caution, but they
may reflect that lesbian mothers may be more motivated as parents and
more likely to carefully plan their child-rearing experiences—mothering is not quite as automatic for a lesbian as for a heterosexual woman,
thus, children are more often planned, wanted, and cherished.

Peer Relations.   Some critics suggest that children of gay and lesbian
parents may be stigmatized by their peers because of their parents' relationships. Green et al. (1986) found no differences in self-perceived
or mother-perceived popularity, and Golombok et al. (1983) found that
the same number of children of heterosexual mothers and lesbian
mothers reported definite or minor problems with peer relations.
Bozett (1988) found that children of gay fathers employed a number of

effective coping strategies with the outside world and reported that their relationships with their fathers were more open and honest than typical father-child relationships. Good relationships with parents can mediate the impact of poor peer relationships, as well as model good skills for peer relationships.

Other-Sex Role Models.   A criticism often aimed at lesbian parenting is that children of lesbian parents would lack male role models. Golombok et al. (1983) found that children of lesbian mothers were more likely to have contact with their fathers than children of divorced heterosexual mothers. Kirkpatrick et al. (1981) found that lesbian mothers had more male friends and relatives involved with their children's lives than did heterosexual mothers. Similarly, gay male couples are criticized for a lack of a maternal role. It appears that "mothering" can be done by men, and "fathering" by women—these are roles, not biological facts and good parenting can be accomplished by single parents of either gender, same-sex couples, and heterosexual couples.

These studies indicate that children are not harmed, and indeed, may even benefit from having same-sex parents. So why do relatively few same-sex couples choose to parent? Benkov (1994) recounted a conversation she once had with a partner:

> *"The world is so homophobic," she said. "What will happen to a child of lesbians?" I reasoned that, as with other prejudices and as we had done, we would help the child develop resilience in the face of bigotry—that although it would take some work, neither the child nor we would bow under. She responded, "You're stronger than I in that way." Those words ushered me in a bewildering sense of guilt. It rose in my throat and silenced me. "You're stronger than I" translated easily to "You're stronger than a child will be." And then, with no one to suggest otherwise, I saw myself inflicting pain on a not-yet-conceived, but nonetheless already treasured child—inflicting pain by the very act of bringing her into the world. . . . Framed this way, the fact that as a lesbian I so longed to nurture a child was in and of itself evidence that I was far too selfish to do so. . . . My conflict between desire and shame in becoming a lesbian mother reflected but one of the many sharp divisions society makes: Lesbians and gay men are on one side, and children and families on the other. (pp. 4–5)*

Thus, internalized homophobia and homophobia interact to make some same-sex couples or single lesbian, gay, or bisexual people fearful and ashamed of parenting desires. Other barriers include the threat of loss of custody of biological children, laws or social service agency policies that do not allow adoption by same-sex couples or lesbian, gay, or bisexual individuals, and lack (or invisibility) of parent role models in lesbian, gay, and bisexual communities. Table 4.2 describes some of the legal battles lesbian, gay, and bisexual families have faced in the United States in recent years.

TABLE 4.2. Significant Events in Family Law for Lesbian, Gay, and Bisexual People

Date	Event
1977	Anita Bryant's "Save the Children" campaign in Florida, where she described homosexuals as human garbage and child molesters, results in a law barring gay adoption.
1978	Senator John Briggs proposes a bill to the California legislature that would ban all gay teachers from public schools—it did not pass.
1985	A Massachusetts gay couple fostering two young children are pushed into news spotlight by a few irate neighbors. The boys are removed from their home and then Governor Dukakis orders a policy review. The policy ultimately becomes so restrictive that single heterosexuals or unmarried couples are also barred (it took 5 years to rescind the policy).
1986	The New Hampshire legislature passes a bill prohibiting gays from foster care, adoption, and day care. Bill sponsor Mildred Ingram said, "I am not against homosexuals. . . . They can go on their merry way to hell if they want. I just want them to keep their filthy paws off the children."
1991	ACLU challenges the Florida law and it is struck down in one county.
1994	Sharon Bottoms loses custody of her child on the basis of social stigma.
Late 1990's	22 states still have sodomy laws, decreasing the likelihood that same-sex couples can adopt in those states, and increasing the chance of loss of custody. Most of Florida and all of New Hampshire still bans gays from adopting; only a few states have laws that ban discrimination on the basis of sexual orientation.

Note. Adapted from Benkov (1994) and Martin (1993).

When lesbian, gay, and bisexual people choose to raise children, they do so for mostly the same reasons as heterosexuals do, and they do not differ dramatically in their attitudes about child-rearing or in parenting styles (Bigner & Jacobsen, 1989a, 1989b), although they may be more likely to teach their children to value diversity and respect others who are different.

The routes to parenting are varied for lesbian, gay, and bisexual people, just as they are for heterosexuals. Lesbians and bisexual women can become parents by traditional heterosexual unions, either in marriage or having sex with a man with the express intention of conceiving, donor insemination (a survey of physicians in 1979 showed that 90% would refuse DI to a lesbian, but this is changing, Benkov, 1994), adoption, and second parent adoption. Gay and bisexual men can become parents through heterosexual unions, such as marriage, through surrogacy arrangements, adoption, and second parent adoptions. Men or women can become foster parents or engage in formal or informal parenting arrangements (e.g., a gay man may provide sperm for the insemination of one of a lesbian couple, then take a godparent role in the child's life).

A major issue in family health care today is that of the blended family and helping children and adults adjust to new family configurations. Lesbian, gay, and bisexual families often face such blendings, and nonbiological, nonlegal parents may have more difficulty defining their roles in the family. There may be different levels of parent-child attachment, depending on biological closeness. The nonbiological parent cannot experience pregnancy, birth, and nursing directly, and may feel shut out. Nonbiological parents have no social validity and are often not recognized as a parent, and most importantly, they lack any legal authority. If a child in the care of a nonbiological parent suddenly falls ill, that parent may not have any authority to make health care decisions.

Coming Out to Children

Another difficult disclosure decision for many lesbian, gay, and bisexual people is when and how to come out to children. In general, research indicates that children who are told at a relatively young age adjust easier than children who are told when they are older (Barrett &

Robinson, 1990). Some parents choose not to disclose to their children in an effort to "protect" them. For example:

> *I knew that my children had not asked to have a father who is gay, and I just could not bring myself to tell them until they became adults. I hoped that by then they would be successfully launched into life and that my lifestyle would have little impact on them. After I first told them, they were really angry with me. Finally two of them have come around and seem to want to be a part of my life. The other two are still somewhat wary and reserved. If I could be 20 again, I would probably still marry and have children, for my life with my wife and kids has been deeply meaningful to me. I would not trade the 28 years with them for anything. (Barrett & Robinson, 1990, pp. 82-83)*

Other parents tell their children early on because they do not want to convey a message of shame or embarrassment about their families but hope instead to strengthen their children with coping mechanisms. Parents should not rely on teachers for support—some will be supportive, others may be uncomfortable, and yet others overtly homophobic. Phyllis Burke (1993) described the changes that she went through when her partner became pregnant and subsequently had a child. Phyllis had to confront homophobia in a different way now that a child was involved—she and her partner had to decide if they would be out and open in all situations, and if they were, how would that affect their child? She became a gay rights activist because of her wish to make the world a safer and better place for her child. Parents who are committed to justice and seek a fair world will convey a message of strength, pride, and integrity to their children.

One child whose lesbian mothers had been honest with her from an early age said:

> *It's both good and bad to be different—you're original, some people react like, you're different, it's cool, so why don't you tell people about your difference? But then it's bad 'cause other people react like you're different from them and they don't want any part of that difference. Some people say, "What do you do at home"—like it's so different. I eat dinner, do my homework—the same things you do. I don't really care anymore. It*

used to bother me. I'd think, I'm not different, am I really dif-
ferent? Why am I different? And I didn't know why—what was
different. Did I do things differently when I went home. . . . It got
me thinking. (Benkov, 1994, pp. 202-203)

This child, who was very accepting of her lesbian mothers when she was young, had more difficulty as she approached her teen years. She became more cautious in selecting friends and rarely brought them to her home; however, when directly faced with homophobia from her peers, she was not afraid to confront it. We need to remember that children are constantly evolving and developing cognitive abilities—as they grow, reactions to family structures may change, just as adults change and evolve in their thinking. Coming out to children often involves more than just disclosure of a parent's sexuality; it may follow or precipitate other family changes such as a divorce or separation. Attitudes of grandparents and other family members may change, and the parent may be experiencing additional stresses of homophobia (e.g., employment) in ways that affect family life.

Unique Problems with Children

The same issues that affect lesbian, gay, and bisexual couples described in the previous section (disclosure to health care providers, violence, living with illness, etc.) also apply to families with children. Unique problems, however, may arise with children. For example, can the non-biological parent make decisions about a child's health care? How do couples decide whether to disclose to the child's pediatrician or teachers at school? Can the coparent be allowed to visit and participate in the child's care or schooling in the same way as a heterosexual parent? How do children deal with their family structure? How do they learn to present the issue to friends? Benkov (1994) suggests that parents need to directly and deliberately teach their children how to address teasing and prepare them for the homophobia that they will eventually encounter in the world. Children with good coping skills often have a high degree of self-confidence. A 5-year-old child in my community informed her kindergarten teacher one day, "Teacher, I don't want to be a tattletale, but Melissa said it's gross to have two mothers. I told her that she was wrong, but she wouldn't listen to me. Will you *please* tell her that she is wrong?"

STRATEGIES FOR HEALTH CARE PROVIDERS

Health care professionals must make a commitment to educate themselves about lesbian, gay, and bisexual issues. Although our socialization is not our fault and we can't help growing up in a homophobic, racist, sexist society, we are responsible for our adult beliefs. While negative attitudes based on inaccurate stereotypes about lesbian, gay, and bisexual people must be replaced with accurate information, changes in individual beliefs alone are not sufficient. Our health care systems reflect the general society in which racism, sexism, and homophobia are deeply embedded. Health care providers can work to make the system safer and more accessible to lesbian and gay families by educating themselves and their coworkers and examining their policies and procedures via continuing education programs, reading, discussion groups, guest speakers, and films.

Health care providers also need to consider current definitions of family. The notion of the traditional family with two parents, one male and one female, who are raising one or more children in their first and only marriage is no longer adequate. Many children now grow up in other family forms—they have single parents who never married, single parents who are separated, divorced, cohabiting, or widowed. They come from blended stepfamilies or are raised by grandparents, siblings, or aunts and uncles. Children are fostered or adopted by strangers, born via donor insemination, and so on. While the old traditional family is touted as "morally superior," child abuse and neglect, alcoholism, and mental illnesses can be found within even those "superior" families. For the sake of your own health care agency, consider broadening your definitions of family and determine what you need to know about the patient or client's family. Then ask relevant questions instead of "Are you married?" Same-sex families can be more complex than the traditional nuclear family (e.g., Barrett & Robinson, 1990, reported eight different configurations of gay father families).

Health care workers have a particular need to know the local resources for lesbian and gay families, such as gay and lesbian organizations and support groups, gay and lesbian affirmative counselors, physicians, lawyers, and religious leaders. They also should be familiar with local hospital, clinic, and social service agencies policies regarding same-sex couples and should find out whether the state or city they live in has a nondiscrimination policy (or human rights policy) that includes sexual orientation. Does the state have sodomy laws that render consensual same-sex sexual behaviors illegal? Do state adoption or foster care laws permit same-sex couples to raise children? What is the hospital policy regarding donor insemination; who is permitted to stay with the mother in the delivery room? Are these policies discriminatory against same-sex couples?

Health care providers need to be accomplished at assessing social support for their clients. Will the client have a supportive partner, family of origin, family of creation, or community to foster recovery? If the client is very "closeted" and without much support, health care providers need to know how to refer the client to services that bolster that support—confidential counseling by a gay-affirmative professional, a support group, a clergy member, and so on.

To protect their relationships, lesbian and gay families need several kinds of legal documents such as wills and power of attorney for finances and health care (see Curry & Clifford, 1991, for a detailed discussion of these documents).[1] Health care providers need to be skilled at evaluating relationships and advising couples on how to protect their relationships, particularly when one of the couple has a chronic illness, or when child custody is threatened. Interviews with new clients should always include information about legal documents. If your agency has a standard form, there should be a space to indicate whether any person holds power of attorney for health care or legal guardianship papers for the client/patient. If so, a copy of these documents should be kept with the client's medical record or chart.

Health care providers also need to recognize the effects of homophobia and heterosexism on the family unit. Some problems may be directly due to societal treatment, not individual shortcomings. If the child of a lesbian couple who is well-behaved at home and has always had good reports from school suddenly begins experiencing negative treatment from a teacher, this may be due to the teacher's homophobia, and is not the fault of the child or the parents. If a gay male father is depressed, it may be due to stresses of the workplace, to rejection by the family of origin, or concern about custody of his child rather than some endogenous chemical imbalance. The bisexual woman who seems defensive and hostile to health care providers may have had bad experiences in the past that have rendered her suspicious.

---

[1]The Appendix contains a sample power of attorney for health care.

Good interviewing techniques and understanding of homophobia are necessary to uncover these problems.

Homophobia is so pervasive in society that health care providers need to be alert to signs of internalized homophobia in a lesbian, gay, or bisexual person such as low self-esteem, shame, or guilt about sexual orientation, increased alcohol and drug use, symptoms of depression, and suicide attempts. Lesbian or gay people with these symptoms may need help from a supportive lesbian, gay, bisexual affirmative professional counselor or a support group.

Health care providers can also help children of same-sex couples in learning stress reduction techniques and coping skills. They may need to practice telling their friends or teachers about their parents, and they may need validation. Some children of lesbian and gay parents may feel isolated because their experiences are not reflected in the books they read at school or the TV programs, magazines, or movies they look at. Children need to be provided with age-appropriate materials that affirm their family structures, such as books, videos, and support groups. Some good resources are listed in Table 4.3.

Some children or adolescents may be questioning their sexual identity, and need educational resources and support while they struggle with their own identity crises. Few school libraries in this conservative climate have such resources, so you may need to find alternative routes for information, such as public libraries and lesbian, gay, and bisexual organizations. More about adolescents and the coming out process will be discussed in Chapter 6.

Health care providers have a responsibility to learn about lesbian and gay families, because they can have a major impact on these family units, depending on their attitudes. Negative attitudes can lead to poor quality of health care, or no health care provision at all. Positive attitudes can lead to good health care and can build rapport with lesbian and gay communities that are distrustful because of previous problems with health care providers.

EXERCISE: "FAMILY VALUES"

Make a mental list of the qualities that you consider to be "good family values." After you have made this list, think about whether any of these qualities are influenced by sexual identity. A widely displayed bumper

TABLE 4.3. Resources for Children and Lesbian, Gay, and Bisexual Parents

Books for Young Children

Bosche, S. (1981). *Jenny lives with Eric and Martin.* London: Gay Men's Press.

Elwin, R. & Paulse, M. (1990). *Asha's mums.* Toronto: Women's Press.

Heron, A., & Maran, M. (1991). *How would you feel if your dad was gay?* Boston: Alyson.

Newman, L. (1989). *Heather has two mommies.* Boston: Alyson.

Wilhoite, M. (1990). *Daddy's roommate.* Boston: Alyson.

Wilhoite, M. (1991). *Families: A coloring book.* Boston: Alyson.

Books for Adolescents

Alyson, S. (Ed.). (1991). *Young, gay, and proud.* Boston: Alyson.

Pollack, R., & Schwartz, C. (1995). *The journey out: A guide for and about lesbian, gay, and bisexual teens.* New York, NY: Viking.

Videos

Sands, A., & Banks, D. (1987). *We are family.* WGBH-TV, 125 Western Ave. Allston, MA, 02134 (617-492-2777).

White, K. (1987). *Not all parents are straight.* Cinema Guild, 1697 Broadway, Suite 802, New York, NY, 10019 (212-246-5522).

Organizations

Gay and Lesbian Parents Coalition International, PO Box 50360, Washington, DC, 20091 (202-583-8029).

Lambda Legal Defense and Education Fund, 666 Broadway, New York, NY, 10012 (212-995-8585).

National Gay and Lesbian Task Force, 1734 14th St., NW, Washington, DC, 20009-4309 (202-332-6483).

Parents and Friends of Lesbians and Gays, 1012 14th St. NW, Suite 700, Washington, DC, 20005 (202-638-4200).

sticker and t-shirt slogan in my area states: "Hatred is not a family value." The sentiment behind the slogan is that the only thing that distinguishes lesbian, gay, and bisexual families from others is societal disapproval and hatred. Imagine that a same-sex couple with three children, aged 2 to 12, moved into your neighborhood. How do you think your neighbors would react? What could you do to make the family feel welcome and safe?

Chapter Five

Health Care Provider Attitudes

Jennie had been experiencing lower abdominal pain and menstrual spotting for two weeks, and finally decided to go to the Student Health Service at the college she attended. She had been there two months earlier for a Pap test but had not disclosed her sexual identity at that time. She had looked carefully at the brochures in the information rack, the posters on the walls, the books in the physician's office, and saw nothing concerning lesbian, gay, or bisexual people. The forms that she had filled out and the interviews by the nurse and physician had not provided any opportunities either. So instead of telling them of her relationship with a woman, she had merely answered "yes" to the question about sexual activity and had endured the ensuing lecture about birth control. Jennie had even taken the prescription for birth control pills that the physician had pressed on her, but tore it up on her way out. The whole experience had been uncomfortable, but given her current marginal employment status, she could not afford to go to a private physician's office, nor did she expect that things would be that much different if she did.

But today she was feeling terrible and felt she had to see a physician—the abdominal pain came in sharp waves that nearly doubled her over. When she was called to the exam room, a very sympathetic nurse took her vital signs and asked why she was there. Jennie must have looked frightened, because the nurse patted her on the shoulder and gave her a comforting smile. "We'll take care of it," she said in reassuring tones, and left to get the physician.

After the physical exam, the physician said, "I believe you might have an ectopic pregnancy. We will need to do a pregnancy test right now and schedule you for an ultrasound this afternoon."

Jennie gulped, then said, "But I can't be pregnant."

The nurse put her hand on Jennie's shoulder and replied in a voice meant to soothe the irrational patient, "The pregnancy test will tell us for sure. You know, birth control pills are not 100% effective."

"No," Jennie insisted, "I'm sure that I'm not pregnant."

Both the nurse and physician looked skeptical—her medical record said that she had been sexually active just two months ago—they obviously suspected denial on her part so Jennie took a deep breath and blurted out, "I can't be pregnant because I am a lesbian. My sexual partner is a woman."

The physician leaned back in her chair, increasing the distance between herself and Jennie, and the nurse, so comforting a moment ago, could not maintain eye contact.

"I see," the physician said finally. "That changes everything. Why didn't you tell us this in the first place?"

Now Jennie felt as if she were being blamed for wasting their valuable time. Eyes downcast, she mumbled, "I didn't know it was relevant."

The nurse and physician left the room, but Jennie could hear them talking in the hallway—she couldn't hear the words, but she could imagine what they were saying. What would happen when they returned? Would they put "lesbian" in big red letters on her medical record? Would they reveal her sexual identity to her academic program in early childhood education? The pain in her abdomen flared again and she clutched her knees in agony. Why didn't she bring Claire along? She could really use some moral support now.

Finally, after nearly 20 minutes, they returned. The nurse remained in the doorway, as the physician stood awkwardly in front of Jennie and said, "We will draw some blood for tests and you will need to give us a urine sample to look for signs of infection." She busied herself preparing Jennie's arm for blood-drawing and she never once looked Jennie in the eye. Jennie noticed that several other staff members walked by the open door and glanced in. Was she the freak of the day? Again she yearned for Claire's support. What was wrong with her? The physician had not offered any possible explanation for the pain and Jennie was afraid to ask. As the physician completed drawing the blood, she handed the tube to the nurse who took it in her gloved hand.

This scenario depicts one of the most common experiences that lesbian, gay, and bisexual people have with health care providers. Although more extreme incidents do occur, like rough physical handling or refusal of care, many lesbian, gay, and bisexual people report this distant, polite, but distinctly chilly approach when they reveal their sexual identity. In this chapter, I will review studies of the attitudes of health care providers toward both homosexuality and AIDS since AIDS and homosexuality became linked in the public mind in the 1980s. I will also describe the perceptions of lesbian, gay, and bisexual people of their health care, the rates of self-disclosure and the ways that some people go about deciding whether to reveal their sexual identity, and finally, the ways that negative attitudes might influence the behavior of health care providers.

ATTITUDES OF HEALTH CARE PROVIDERS

Most health care providers are still socialized within the "equal treatment" model; that is, all clients/patients deserve the same treatment regardless of any human characteristics such as race, ability to pay, religion, or social class. Sexual identity, however, seems to be exempt from the model, as very little literature has been devoted to understanding the needs of lesbian, gay, and bisexual clients/patients. Prior to college and sometimes even in school, most health care providers are socialized to believe that same-sex relationships are deviant, sinful, unusual, "exotic," and/or inferior to heterosexual relationships. Since their health care education rarely challenges these stereotypes or presents factual information about lesbian, gay, and bisexual clients, these negative attitudes are often reflected in their practice. Even if health care providers seek information on their own, what do their professional journals or health-oriented textbooks tell them?

Prior to the 1970s, most articles and books on homosexuality in health care libraries reflected the still popular viewpoint of homosexuality as mental illness. In 1964, for example, the highly regarded journal *RN* printed an article entitled, "Understanding the Homosexual Patient"

(Juzwiak, 1964), which attempted to take an "enlightened" view, but comes off as quite offensive today. The author noted that with increased visibility of homosexuality in society, "the nurse is more likely to find herself caring for patients who are known or suspected sexual deviates" (p. 53). And the suggestions for nurses are sexist as well as homophobic:

> *The female nurse dealing with a homosexual patient ought to avoid behavior that, while potentially pleasing to a heterosexual male, might be irritating or seem threatening to the homosexual male. Specifically, she should avoid being flirtatious with him, or unduly "pressuring." (p. 57)*
>
> *The male nurse or attendant working with a male homosexual patient should bear in mind the possibility that normal friendly and solicitous behavior might be misinterpreted. (p. 57)*
>
> *Certainly, the degree to which she is able to view the homosexual person as a human being with a special problem rather than as an unspeakable and frightening "pervert" will not only help her to work with such patients but will also beneficially influence the attitudes of other hospital personnel who come into contact with them. (p. 118)*

This type of article did little to dispel negative stereotypes or improve the health care of the homosexual patient. But by the mid-1970s, the tone of many articles began to change. Lawrence (1975), writing as a gay man, exhorted nurses to treat gay patients with respect and dignity and noted, "Nurses' failure to recognize the depth, variety, and meaning of homosexual lifestyles can be a constant source of distress to homosexual patients" (p. 307). Instead of blaming the patient for behaviors that may distress nurses, he puts the blame on nurses, concluding, "To endure a hospital stay may be one of the most bitter and unpleasant of any of the oppressive experiences that homosexual persons are subject to daily" (p. 308).

Brossart (1979) insisted that prejudiced nurses would give poor care:

> *"What's the difference if the patient is gay? It's none of my business. And I wouldn't want to pry." "I treat everyone the same way, anyhow." At first glance, these statements might seem to reflect an enlightened attitude toward the treatment of the homosexual patient. But beware. The first could lead toward a life-threatening situation for your patient. And the second is probably not even true. (p. 51)*

From these early opinion-based articles criticizing nurses' negative attitudes, the first empirically based research studies of health care provider attitudes began to emerge, though in tandem with the opinion pieces for a time. Although attitudes might have steadily improved over the years as more research revealed that homosexuals are not mentally ill and do not differ from heterosexuals on nearly any personality measure, the AIDS epidemic, which started in the 1980s, proved a setback for the battle against prejudicial attitudes. In a 1984 letter to the editor of the *Southern Medical Journal,* a physician asserted:

> *A strange disorder with a strange predilection is AIDS. Why? . . . Might we be witnessing, in fact, in the form of a modern communicable disorder, a fulfillment of St. Paul's pronouncement: "the due penalty of their error?" . . . Might it be that our society's approval of homosexuality is an error and that the unsubtle words of wisdom of the Bible are frightfully correct? (Fletcher, 1984, p. 149)*

Schwanberg (1990) reviewed the health care literature from 1974 to 1987. Dividing the time period into pre-AIDS (1975–1983) and post-AIDS (1983–1987), she found more negative images of lesbians and gay men in the more recent literature than in the older. In 1975–1983, she found 57 articles, 16 of which portrayed lesbians and gay men in a negative way. In 1983–1987, she found 59 articles, 36 of which had negative images (and only six of which were positive portrayals). Have these negative portrayals of lesbian, gay, and bisexual people in the health care literature reinforced the negative stereotypes that health care providers learn in the culture at large?

A recent Gallup poll found that 53% of Americans believed that "homosexual lifestyles" are unacceptable, 45% thought that gay rights are a threat to the American family and its values, and 49% said that homosexuals should not be employed as elementary school teachers. Additionally, 58% were opposed to legalizing marriage for same-sex partners, and 61% were against adoption rights for lesbian, gay, and bisexual people (Turque, 1992).

Although it might seem natural for health care providers to be more caring individuals, thus less likely to have prejudices and more likely to be open-minded, there is little research supporting that claim. Our culture exposes us to prejudicial attitudes and behavior early on, and only by learning accurate information and directly confronting our own prejudices can we overcome this negative training. Health care education rarely provides this essential information about lesbian and gay clients to counteract the stereotypes (Randall, 1987).

Stevens (1992) provided a review of 20 years of research on health care provider attitudes about lesbians, citing 28 studies. Nine involved health care provider attitudes about lesbians and 19 chronicled lesbians' perceptions of their own health care. Gay men and bisexuals of either sex have not been studied as extensively, though it is likely that the same general findings apply. A few of these studies are reviewed in the following sections.

Surveys of Health Care Providers about Their Attitudes

White (1979) distributed questionnaires to 67 psychiatric nurses (62 women and 5 men). The two forms of the survey included the Attitudes toward Homosexuality Scale (ATHS) and a scenario about two psychiatric patients who began to spend much time together and sought out privacy. In one form the two patients are a woman and a man, and in the other form, the two patients are both women. The nurses answered questions about the relationship (whether they just enjoyed each other's company and sought privacy for conversation, whether they were seeking physical contact, whether they were seeking sexual contact and cared about each other, or whether they sought sex without caring for each other) and the appropriateness of the relationship (inappropriate because of being patients, inappropriate in any setting, a manifestation of their psychopathology, an appropriate relationship, inappropriate only because of excluding other patients). White found that negative attitudes were quite prevalent and that greater negativity was related to religion and education. Catholics and Protestants were more negative than atheists, and those who considered themselves to be "devout" or moderately religious were more negative than those whose faith was "inactive." Education had a positive effect on attitudes, with greater education related to more positive attitudes on the ATHS. Responses to the scenario showed that nurses were likely to attribute desire for physical closeness to a heterosexual couple, but attribute a desire for conversation to two women, thus denying the possibility of physical intimacy between women. More nurses rated the same-sex scenario as inappropriate for any reason (44%) than the opposite-sex scenario (33%).

Douglas, Kalman, and Kalman (1985) surveyed 37 physicians and 91 nurses from a large urban teaching hospital that provided AIDS care to many patients. They found, contrary to most other studies, that the women were more homophobic than the men. Having a close friend or family member who was homosexual led to more positive attitudes. About one-third of the physicians and nurses agreed that AIDS patients received inferior care compared with other patients, and 3% of physicians and 12% of nurses believed, "Homosexuals who contract AIDS are getting what they deserve." Over 30% of the sample agreed that they had more negative attitudes about homosexuality since the AIDS epidemic began.

Matthews, Booth, Turner, and Kessler (1986) surveyed physicians from the San Diego County Medical Society. They obtained a response rate of 43%, with over 1,000 respondents on a questionnaire that included the Heterosexuals Attitudes toward Homosexuality Scale (HATH: Larsen, Reed, & Hoffman, 1980). Respondents were 93% male and primarily in private practice (86%) or academic medicine (11%). Table 5.1 summarizes some of their results, showing that women had more favorable attitudes than men and that physicians in academic settings had more favorable attitudes than those in private practice. In addition, more recent graduation from medical school was associated with more favorable attitudes.

By specialty, the three most positive (ones with highest percentage of favorable responses) were psychiatry, pediatrics, and internal medicine. The specialties with the highest number of members with negative attitudes were orthopedic surgery, obstetrics and gynecology, and general and family practice. The latter two specialities are likely to

TABLE 5.1. Heterosexual Attitudes toward Homosexuals (HATH) Scores by Sex and Setting

HATH Score	Overall (%)	Women (%)	Men (%)	Private Practice (%)	Academic (%)
Favorable	37	51	36	33	59
Neutral	40	23	41	41	28
Unfavorable	34	26	24	26	13

Note. Adapted from Matthews, Booth, Turner, and Kessler (1986).

have high numbers of lesbian, gay, and bisexual clients. On other attitudinal questions, the authors found that nearly 30% were opposed to admitting highly qualified homosexual applicants to medical school, 45% were opposed to homosexual physicians training in pediatrics, and more than 40% would stop referring patients to a pediatrician or psychiatrist on learning the physician was homosexual. Finally, over 39% reported that they were sometimes or often uncomfortable when treating homosexual patients. This finding suggests that the HATH scores may underestimate negative attitudes, since only 23% of respondents were rated as having unfavorable attitudes on the HATH, yet 39% reported feeling uncomfortable when caring for homosexual patients.

Young (1988) surveyed 22 registered nurses who were attending a workshop on AIDS, and found that 64% entered with negative attitudes about homosexuals, expressed in terms such as pity, disgust, discomfort, and repulsion. Over half of the sample initially saw no need or desire to change their negative attitudes, illustrating the difficulty achieving change if a substantial number of people are not motivated to change, or even to challenge, their current thinking.

Randall (1989) examined the responses of 100 midwestern nurse educators on questions about lesbians and health care. A large number reported negative attitudes about lesbians in general. For example, 52% agreed that lesbianism is unnatural (this finding parallels the 1992 *Newsweek* poll, which found that 53% thought homosexuality is unacceptable), 34% agreed that lesbianism is "disgusting," or immoral (23%), 17% thought lesbianism is a disease, and another 17% thought that lesbians molest children. Regarding health care practice, 4% said that they would refuse to care for a lesbian, and 13% did not want a lesbian nurse to care for them. Nursing education rarely covered lesbian issues in the clinical setting or the lecture room. Over 50% had never discussed lesbian issues in the classroom and 28% were uncomfortable with the idea of teaching about lesbian clients. Only 10% routinely included discussion of lesbians in their clinical settings, and 18% said they included it in their lectures. Ten percent thought that lesbians should not be allowed to teach in schools of nursing. Finally, 20% thought that lesbians were a common source of HIV transmission. These educators most likely convey their negative attitudes and misconceptions to their students.

Chaimowitz (1991) surveyed 72 physicians who were psychiatric residents, staff psychiatrists, and family practice residents at a medical school in Ontario. Family practice residents were more likely to be ho-mophobic (36%) than staff (26%) or resident psychiatrists (33%). Men were significantly more homophobic than women (40% compared with 14%). Like the Matthews et al. (1986) study previously cited, many family practice physicians were found to be homophobic.

Eliason and Randall (1991) studied attitudes of 120 female nursing students regarding lesbians. The questionnaire included information about the students' backgrounds, their current attitudes, the Bem Sex-Role Inventory, and a brief scenario about a lesbian. Respondents received one of two forms that differed only by the photograph that accompanied the scenario. In one form, the photograph showed a woman in "feminine" attire—a dress and dress shoes. In the other form, the same woman wore "nonfeminine" attire—jeans and hiking boots. Respondents were asked questions about their likelihood of having social contact with this woman, the physical attractiveness of the woman, and their attitudes and knowledge about lesbians. A control group of students had previously rated the photos for physical attractiveness and no differences were found for the feminine and nonfeminine pictures when sexual identity was not known. When the woman was labeled as a lesbian, however, she was rated as significantly less attractive in nonfeminine attire. Twenty-six percent of the respondents said that lesbians were unacceptable and that they would avoid all contact with a lesbian. Nearly 30% thought that lesbians were a high-risk group for AIDS. Ratings on the Bem Sex-Role Inventory (feminine, masculine, androgynous, or undifferentiated) did not predict attitudes about lesbians.

Eliason, Donelan, and Randall (1992) conducted a content analysis of written comments from 189 female nursing students, some of whom had participated in the preceding study. The major themes that emerged were representative of common stereotypes about lesbians. The most common theme was a fear of seduction. Of these respondents, 38% were concerned that lesbian coworkers or patients might try to "hit on" them, and 29% thought that lesbians tried to "push their beliefs" on others by "flaunting" their sexuality. One respondent noted, "I would hope this type of woman would respect me and others and not talk about her lifestyle freely." Over 30% thought that lesbians could be identified by their masculine appearance. A significant minority of nursing students objected to lesbians on moral or religious grounds (13%) or biological unnaturalness, such as the perceived inability to procreate (14%). Another 11% thought that lesbians were poor role models for children.

Harris, Nightengale, and Owen (1995) surveyed 97 health care providers (nurses, social workers, and psychologists) about their knowledge, experience, and attitudes about homosexuality. Among the 97 respondents, 9% were lesbian, gay, or bisexual. Respondents were presented with a case study of a fictitious client where the genders of the client and the client's lover were varied. Respondents had to rate their attitudes about working with the client, and provide a tentative diagnosis. There were no significant differences on the measures by gender of the client or client's lover. Next, the respondents described their experiences with homosexuality. As a group, they had spent an average of 3.3 classroom hours in their academic programs on homosexuality, although 51% reported that they never had any content on homosexuality in school. The majority felt that more time needed to be devoted to these issues (94%), and indeed 74% had attended workshops to supplement their knowledge. Social workers expressed a greater need for training than did nurses. Respondents said that their beliefs about homosexuality were shaped by their personal experiences (69%), their personal beliefs (51%), their work experiences (21%), educational experiences (11%), and religion (8%). Twenty percent condoned discrimination on the basis of sexual orientation. Female psychologists and male social workers had more positive attitudes about working with lesbian, gay, or bisexual clients than did the other groups. Although these respondents had generally higher scores (e.g., were less homophobic) on the homophobia measure than college students (reported in studies by Herek, 1988), nurses were more homophobic as a group than social workers or psychologists. Nurses also had lower scores on the knowledge test. Of the three groups, however, nurses had the lowest level of education, a variable found to correlate with knowledge about homosexuality. In general, the more knowledgeable respondents were less prejudiced.

All these studies indicate that a significant number of health care providers have negative attitudes about lesbian, gay, and bisexual people. They also suggest a lack of knowledge about homosexuality, and some studies find a link between lack of knowledge and prejudice. Since the early 1980s, however, these attitudes have changed somewhat because of AIDS.

Attitudes about AIDS and Homosexuality: A Deadly Interaction

Attitudes about AIDS also influence health care providers' care of lesbian, gay, and bisexual people. Negative attitudes may have increased in response to AIDS, as lesbian, gay, and bisexual people were blamed for bringing AIDS to the general population (Alexander & Fitzpatrick, 1990; Schwanberg, 1990). Attitudes about AIDS represent two distinct but overlapping kinds of fear (Herek & Glunt, 1988). The first, AIDS-related stigma, involves the difficulties our society has with death and dying, compounded by the fear of contagion. Although this fear was more reasonable in earlier years when knowledge about the virus was limited, some health care providers continue to have an irrational fear of transmission. In one study, for example, nursing students wrote: "I feel that because of my actual fear of contracting AIDS, I could not care for AIDS patients the way they deserve. I would be weary [sic] of close physical contact" and "I am too scared of contracting the AIDS virus from the patient's urine" (Eliason, 1993a, p. 29). The fear of death and dying is pervasive in our society and is magnified in young health care providers who care for dying patients no older than themselves.

The second fear is related to homophobia and lack of experience working with gay or bisexual clients. Regarding this fear, nursing students wrote: "I do not approve of homosexuals and don't feel I could have compation [sic] for someone who got AIDS due to homosexual practices" and "I totally disagree with these lifestyles because of my morals that I have and was brought up with" (Eliason, 1993a, p. 29). The remainder of this section will examine studies that focus on the intersection of homophobia and AIDS phobia.

O'Donnell et al. administered questionnaires and interviews to 237 hospital employees who worked with AIDS patients (O'Donnell, O'Donnell, Pleck, Snarey, & Rose, 1987). Questions included their knowledge and attitudes about AIDS, attitudes about homosexuality, and the stresses associated with AIDS care. The sample contained professional and technical health care providers, 67% of whom were women. Nearly one-half were nurses, 19% technicians, 14% physicians, 11% LPNs or orderlies, and 8% social workers and clergy. Only 60% thought they had enough information to work effectively with AIDS patients, a lack of knowledge that was reflected in their overestimates of HIV infection rates in gay men and the belief that casual contact could transmit HIV.

The majority (over 73%) agreed that AIDS had made them think more about homosexuality, and nearly 20% said that they were more negative about homosexuality since AIDS. Only 18% had become more "tolerant" of homosexuality. Although most respondents believed that homosexuals deserved basic civil rights (80%), only 36% thought that homosexuality was a natural expression of love. Nearly half of the sample found the thought of homosexual acts disgusting, and 43% said that if their child showed homosexual tendencies, they would want to obtain psychiatric help for her/him. People who were homophobic were also AIDS-phobic and experienced greater stress about AIDS care.

In another study, 119 second- and third-year medical students were presented with four vignettes about a young man named Mark, who was a successful, outgoing, athletic college graduate who had been experiencing fatigue, malaise, and recurrent infections (Kelly, Lawrence, Smith, Hood, and Cook, 1987). Mark was described as either having AIDS or leukemia, and as having a long-term romantic partner named Robert or Roberta. Students gave more negative responses when the condition was AIDS and when the patient was gay. They were significantly more likely to indicate that AIDS patients were responsible for their own illnesses, deserved what they got, should be quarantined, deserved to lose their jobs, and deserved to die. Students were also very likely to indicate that they would have virtually no social contact with an AIDS patient or a homosexual.

Fish and Rye (1991) gave 120 undergraduate students (mean age of about 20) a questionnaire measuring their attitudes and knowledge of AIDS, and one of eight written descriptions accompanying the same picture of a moderately attractive White male. The target male, "Bill," was labeled as homosexual or heterosexual, and as healthy, having terminal cancer, having a venereal disease, or having AIDS. Respondents then rated Bill on likability, morality, intelligence, promiscuity, and other personal characteristics, as well as rating their own likelihood of interacting with Bill. Male respondents gave more unfavorable ratings when Bill was labeled as homosexual than did female respondents. Knowledge about AIDS did not affect the results much—Bill was rated more negatively when labeled as homosexual for all four health conditions. The authors pointed out that knowledge alone is insufficient to change deeply ingrained negative attitudes about homosexuality. Several studies have found that students are more sympathetic to AIDS patients who are not homosexual or IV drug users (Alexander &

Fitzpatrick, 1990; Eliason, 1993a; Lester & Beard, 1988; Meisenhelder & La Charite, 1989; Wells, 1987), thus supporting the interaction of homophobia and AIDS phobia.

EXPERIENCES OF LESBIAN, GAY, AND BISEXUAL PEOPLE WITH HEALTH CARE PROVIDERS

Studies that ask lesbian, gay, and bisexual people about their experiences with health care generally focus on two related topics: whether lesbian, gay, and bisexual people have disclosed their sexual identity to a health care provider, and how the health care provider reacted to discovering or suspecting the client's sexual identity. The following sections describe these issues.

Disclosure of Sexual Identity to Health Care Providers

A respondent in a study of lesbians and health care noted:

> *Lesbians don't say everything that is going on with us. We only give enough information to get what we need from a doctor. We have to protect ourselves. There is always the chance that doctors will treat us differently because we're lesbian, you know, dismiss us, be less concerned, get rough. (Stevens, 1994, p. 223)*

Lesbians (and gay men and bisexuals) may not divulge their sexual identity. The person's dilemma over whether or not to provide this information is complex and stressful in any setting; disclosure to health care providers can be particularly anxiety-provoking. Studies have reported that many lesbian, gay, and bisexual people choose not to reveal their identity, because they fear unpleasant or even life-threatening consequences. Still, nondisclosure is uncomfortable for most people as well and can create feelings of dishonesty, low self-esteem, and lack of personal integrity (Wells & Kline, 1987). Table 5.2 lists some of the studies that have examined rates of disclosure to health care providers, and I will discuss a few of these studies in more detail.

Dardick and Grady (1980) sent questionnaires to the subscribers of the *Gay Community News,* obtaining a sample of 622 respondents who

TABLE 5.2.   Disclosure Rates to Health Care Providers in Samples of
Lesbian, Gay, and Bisexual People

Authors (Year)	Sample	% Who Disclosed
McGhee & Owen (1980)	585 lesbian, gay, & bisexual people	73
Dardick & Grady (1980)	491 gay men	63
Dardick & Grady (1980)	131 lesbians	49
Reagan (1981)	38 lesbians	59
Johnson, Guenther, Laube, & Keettel (1981)	117 lesbians	18
Smith, Johnson, & Guenther (1985)	1921 lesbians, 424 bisexual women	41
Cochran & Mays (1988)	529 black lesbians, 65 black bisexual women	33
Harvey, Carr, & Bernheine (1989)	35 lesbian mothers	91
Zeidenstein (1990)	20 lesbians	50
Eliason & Morgan (1996c)	101 lesbians	59

were primarily male (73%), White (91%), young (78% were between ages 22 and 41), and urban (68%). Nearly three-fourths of the sample had a college degree. The authors reported that 49% had disclosed their sexual identity to a health care provider (63% of the men and 49% of the women), and another 11% assumed that the provider knew. About one-third indicated that they would disclose if it seemed important, and only 7% said they would not disclose under any circumstances. The respondents who had disclosed reported more satisfaction with their health care provider, better communication and, for men, an increased likelihood of receiving a venereal disease checkup. Factors that contributed to disclosure included being open with family and peers, being exclusively or predominantly homosexual, and perceiving the health care provider as supportive.

Many lesbians choose not to disclose their sexual identity (Cochran & Mays, 1988; Deevy, 1993; Hitchcock & Wilson, 1992). As one respondent put it, "I'd probably not bring up my sexual identity unless I saw it as relevant. I don't want to trigger homophobia needlessly when I'm sick" (Eliason & Morgan, 1996c). This quote makes it clear that the respondent expected her disclosure to cause problems. This is not an unrealistic fear—Johnson and Palermo (1984) found that 40% of their predominantly White lesbian respondents expected that disclosure would result in poor treatment, and only 18% had revealed their identity to a physician. Cochran and Mays (1988) found that only about one-third of African American lesbian and bisexual women had self-disclosed to a physician. More recent studies find a slightly higher degree of disclosure, possibly reflecting some changes in societal attitudes. For example, Eliason and Morgan (1996c) found that 65% of lesbians with a regular physician had disclosed their identity.

Hitchcock and Wilson (1992) developed a model for understanding the disclosure process in lesbians (this model likely would apply for gay men and bisexuals as well). They interviewed 33 lesbians aged 18–68 about their health care experiences and found that the process of disclosure had two phases. In the first anticipatory phase, the lesbian imagined what might transpire in the health care setting and used cognitive strategies such as formalizing (giving legal validity to her relationship via power of attorney or other means) and scouting out (collecting information about the health care provider in advance). This anticipatory phase prepared the lesbian for the actual situation, putting her into the interactional phase. When actually faced with the health care provider, the lesbian used strategies such as scanning (observing the setting for any signs of acceptance) and, in the case of a disclosure, monitoring the response of the health care provider. Figure 5.1 shows this model in some detail, adapting Hitchcock and Wilson's model to focus on the two dimensions that impact the disclosure decision; the client and the health care setting (including individual health care provider characteristics). Some dimensions from Stevens's (1994) discussion of lesbian self-protective strategies have been added to the model as well. The complex event of disclosure is a stressor that heterosexual clients do not have, and that health care providers may not have considered.

Lesbian, Gay, and Bisexual People's Perceptions of Their Health Care

Stevens and Hall (1988) found that lesbians had often experienced negative reactions from their health care providers ranging from a condescending attitude, to disapproval, avoidance, and even rough physical handling. They interviewed 25 midwestern lesbians (ages 21–58, with a mean age of 30) about their interactions with health care providers. Approximately 50% of the women in this sample thought that they were

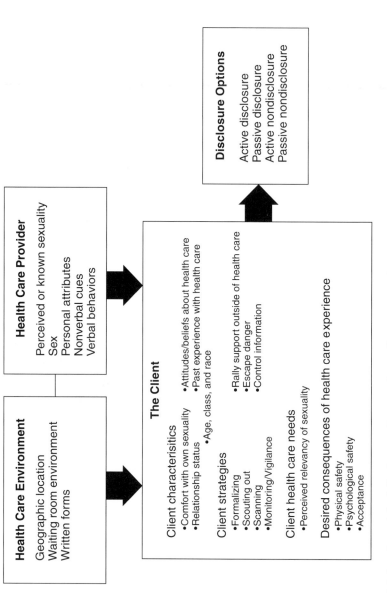

FIGURE 5.1. A model of disclosure: Factors that influence revealing sexual identity to a health care provider. Adapted from Hitchcock & Wilson (1992) and Stevens (1994).

readily identifiable to others as lesbians—only 20% thought that no one could tell by looking at them. Here are some of the reactions that the respondents reported (all quotes from p. 72):

As soon as I said I was a lesbian, the nurses started giving me disgusted looks. They were nasty to my partner. They rough-housed me. They were not gentle like they would be to a straight woman. They treated me like I was "one of those," like they might catch something.

One of the doctors I told turned completely different colors. He left the office saying he had to get equipment and returned with two nurses like he had to have protection from me.

When you go for a Pap test, they always ask if you are sexually active. If you say no, they don't believe you. If you say yes, you get badgered about how you should use birth control. If you are stuck with the birth control lecture, you disclose just to avoid all that. But I've never done it voluntarily. I've always felt forced to disclose.

Virtually all (96%) of the women anticipated situations in which disclosure could have harmful effects, and this anticipation was generally based on negative experiences in the past from health care providers, or from other areas of life:

Society says it's not okay to be a lesbian. We face rejection based on that all the time. Not having access to health care in which it is safe to disclose is just one small part of the larger picture.

If the environment isn't safe for disclosure, I'm not going to be taken care of. I might even get hurt.

It would be very damaging if you got into interactions with health care providers in which you are considered deviant. Some people have very negative, very violent reactions. I don't think they can separate from their personal prejudices. It is like putting your life in someone's hands who really hates you.

Dardick and Grady (1980) found that 35% of respondents who had disclosed their sexual identity found their health care providers to be unsupportive and hostile. About one-fourth of the sample reported they had health-related topics they wished to discuss but felt that they could not because of staff attitudes. Nearly 30% had a past experience with a provider who was prejudiced.

Reagan (1981) asked 38 lesbians what kind of reactions they would expect from health care providers, should they disclose. Fifty percent expected curiosity, 40% thought that disclosure would make the health care provider anxious, and 32% expected that the health care provider would refer them to a psychologist. Nearly 25% of these women had delayed seeking health care when they needed it because of these negative expectations and past experiences.

Geddes (1994) asked 53 lesbians to complete questionnaires about their health care experiences. Most of the respondents relied on family doctors for concerns about health (76%), but 24% would seek advice from other lesbians, friends, or relatives before going to a doctor. Three-fourths of the respondents felt that family physicians were positive and accepting to some degree. When asked to rank the factors they considered important in choosing a family doctor, most said that the doctor's open and receptive manner was the most important (58%). Although 62% preferred female physicians, 34% had no preference, and most in actuality had male physicians. Sixty-five percent had come out to their current physician, but 32% had directly denied their sexual orientation to a physician at some time, mostly out of fear of discrimination (33%). Of the respondents who had not come out to their physician, 89% wanted to. Very few physicians had asked directly about sexual orientation (only 8%), but many had used sex-neutral terms such as partner instead of spouse, indicating some awareness of nonheterosexual relationships (40%). The majority of respondents (92%) thought that it was important to come out to their doctors, not just for the sake of honesty, but so that they would receive accurate diagnoses and treatments and their partners would be included in health care decisions. Geddes found that 19% of respondents who came out to their physician had a negative experience:

[He] interpreted the stress and related depression I was feeling from a new demanding job to my sexual orientation [and] referred me to a psychiatrist.

He asked me if I was married. When I said, "No, I live with my lesbian lover," he was quite embarrassed. Then he told me not to be embarrassed.

During a [second] visit, he again asked me questions about birth control so I had to come out a second time, which was awkward and stressful. This made me even more reluctant to go see a doctor than I already am. (Geddes, 1994, p. 916)

Rose (1993) surveyed 44 lesbian nurses (ranging from students to nurse educators), aged 19–54 years. The majority had been practicing nursing for 6–10 years. One-fourth of the sample was not out to anyone at work, and 50% of those who did come out said that it had been very difficult. Students were less likely than the more mature nurses to come out, because they feared discrimination in the form of bad grades or difficulty finding a job. Many had witnessed discriminatory acts by their nurse colleagues; 25% had experienced another nurse refusing to care for a gay patient. One nurse commented, "I have experienced other nurses/doctors refusing to give a gay man a painkilling suppository in case 'he enjoyed it.' Also, symptoms such as pain being expressed by a gay man were doubted simply because he was gay" (p. 51). All 44 respondents had heard coworkers make derogatory comments about lesbian, gay, or bisexual people.

Related to the findings of Rose's study, Sharon Deevy (1993) reported on her own experiences as a lesbian health care provider:

When I moved to Ohio in 1978 to begin nursing education, I was warned by heterosexual nurses and physicians I knew back in Washington, DC, that an open lesbian could not be a nurse. . . . So after seven years of being out at work as a file clerk, I became a closeted nursing student. The sudden reversal to a double life was jolting, because it takes different sets of skills, compromises, and self-justifications to live either openly or in the closet. . . . During the two years that followed, I was selectively open. I was accepted by many faculty and most students, although each group told me they thought the other group would eventually drive me from the nursing profession. After nursing school, however, I became more secretive again, because I was afraid of losing my new career. In each of my work settings, I saw gay and lesbian patients laughed at, mistreated, or denied. I was effectively intimidated by medical, nursing, and social work colleagues who challenged my tentative efforts at lesbian and gay patient advocacy. Once, at a team conference, I suggested referring a patient to local gay community resources. The psychiatrist refused, and the social worker

*said, glaring at me, "I notice you make that suggestion fre-
quently." Needless to say, I didn't make the suggestion again
soon. (pp. 21-22)*

Deevy offers many helpful tips to lesbian nurses who wish to disclose to coworkers and supervisors and even provides helpful come-
backs to common homophobic comments. Deevy urges lesbian, gay,
and bisexual health care providers to consider being open about themselves at work and cites the positive effects on her own personal and
professional life:

*First, blatant homophobic remarks rarely occur in my presence.
I know they are still made, but the stress of direct homophobic
harassment is gone. Second, I have not been fired. In fact, I have
a greater sense of safety than I did before I disclosed. . . . I feel
an enormous sense of relief now that I no longer lead a double
life. I am energetic, relaxed, and funny in situations in which I
once was secretive and stressed. I have experienced the joy of
being what I yearned to find for myself—a role model as a lesbian nurse. . . . I have learned that there are many heterosexual
nurses who hide their own wisdom about gay and lesbian
culture. Those who have gay and lesbian siblings, children, or
friends have also been hesitant to challenge the bigotry of their
less knowledgeable colleagues. . . . I have seen a great improve-
ment in the nursing care of lesbian and gay patients on my
unit, because my colleagues are comfortable and well-informed
about lesbian and gay culture. . . . I have also learned how
much I had internalized the homophobia of the world around
me. I had not realized how much, as closeted lesbian nurses, we
assume that paranoia, hypervigilance, and lack of spontaneity
at work are inevitable. I also had not realized how we deprive
one another, our patients, and our heterosexual colleagues of
healthy role models. (p. 24)*

Rose and Platzer (1993) conducted a workshop about gay patients, attended primarily by lesbian, gay, and bisexual nurses. They gave many
examples of discriminatory care, including a gay man's chart that was labeled "high risk" simply because he was gay; health care providers in a
genito-urinary clinic who labeled all gay men's specimens with HIV status, while specimens from presumably heterosexual men were not labeled; and the refusal to allow the partner of a lesbian in labor to attend

the delivery. When not overtly discriminatory, lesbian, gay, and bisexual patients were still treated differently:

Even though nurses often declared that they would avoid a lesbian patient or colleague, it was noted that when patients were known to be lesbian, many nurses went out of their way to "have a look" at such women. Such behavior represents unprofessional voyeurism. (Rose & Platzer, 1993, p. 53)

Finally, Stevens (1994) interviewed 45 lesbians about their health care experiences. The women varied widely in racial, ethnic, and economic class status but 77% described their interactions with health care providers as negative, using terms such as "terrified," "betrayed," "traumatized," "unsafe," and "vulnerable." One woman noted:

Lesbians of color are doubly and triply vulnerable when it comes to getting health care. We have to anticipate abuse on so many levels. Structural racism is rampant in health care. Public health services for medically indigent adults are thoroughly inadequate. Doctors and nurses make dangerous and unintelligent responses to lesbians. So we live in double and triple binds that impact our health. It is not safe for us to get health care, so by the time lesbians of color seek services, we are in the last stages of diseases. (Stevens, 1994, p. 220)

Stevens found that lesbians developed a set of eight self-protective strategies for dealing with health care:

1. *Rallying Support.* Turn to friends for help instead of health care providers.
2. *Screening.* Carefully select health care providers if she can afford to do so.
3. *Seeking Mirrors of One's Experience.* Seeking providers who are similar in some ways—lesbians, women, people of color, speak the same language. This is available only to women who can afford to select health care providers.
4. *Maintaining Vigilance.* Scan environment, watch health care providers' reactions.
5. *Controlling Information.* Disclose only if absolutely necessary.

6. *Bringing a Witness.* Avoid being alone with a health care provider.

7. *Challenging Mistreatment.* Negotiate, register a complaint, demand rights.

8. *Escaping Danger.* Leave if feeling threatened.

POTENTIAL BEHAVIORAL CONSEQUENCES OF NEGATIVE ATTITUDES

Homophobia, or the more overtly negative attitudes about lesbian, gay, and bisexual people, will often result in poor quality health care or denial of health care. The negative behaviors of the homophobic health care provider can include avoidance of the gay/lesbian patient, unnecessary referrals for psychiatric consultation, refusal to care for a patient, derogatory comments, and physical mishandling. These experiences create an atmosphere of fear and intimidation for the lesbian, gay, or bisexual client.

Heterosexism has more subtle manifestations, including a condescending attitude, grudging tolerance, and a tendency to treat lesbian and gay clients as wayward children who need the help and protection of the health care provider. These attitudes, though not as dangerous as homophobic reactions, make the health care interaction uncomfortable, and may still impact health care delivery. The incidence of these manifestations of homophobia and heterosexism has yet to be systematically studied, but several studies cited in this chapter provide ample evidence that discriminatory health care practices are widespread. The consequences of discriminatory care can be severe.

One consequence for lesbian, gay, and bisexual clients is that they are often reluctant to seek health care. Stevens and Hall (1988) found that this was true for 84% of the lesbians in their study. Reagan (1981) found that 25% of her sample had delayed getting health care when they needed it. This hesitancy was sometimes from negative past experiences, and sometimes from the expectation that the interaction would be negative or uncomfortable.

Trippet and Bain (1993) surveyed 503 self-identified lesbians about their physical health. The sample was mostly White (93%), young (49% were under 40), and well-educated (76% had a college degree). The lesbians in this sample were most likely to seek health care interventions for menstrual problems, sexually transmitted diseases (mostly vaginal infections), and other reproductive system problems. Many women, however, used self-care or homeopathic remedies rather than formal health care interventions. Several had bad experiences with health care systems and 22% said their health care delivery had been poor or terrible, prompting them to seek alternative treatment.

If lesbian, gay, and bisexual health care providers are known or suspected to be gay, they often face hostility or avoidance from their coworkers. One student in Rose's study (1993) stated, "You know when someone has heard that you're gay because they just change—it's a quick hello, no conversation" (p. 51). Thirty of the 44 lesbian nurses felt the need to censor themselves in breaktime social conversations and 25 of the 44 were afraid to challenge antigay remarks of their colleagues. As Rose noted, both incidents contribute to the "conspiracy of silence" imposed on lesbian, gay, and bisexual health care providers, who ironically, could help educate their coworkers but are often too afraid of workplace or social discrimination to disclose their sexual identities.

CONCLUSION

When researchers ask lesbian, gay, and bisexual people what needs to be changed in health care, the most common response is to reduce the negative attitudes of health care providers. Many lesbian, gay, and bisexual people are afraid to compromise their health care by disclosing their sexual identity; many others, who do disclose, add the stress of disclosure to the stress of illness. A significant number of lesbian, gay, and bisexual people avoid health care altogether. After pointing out the need for changes in individual health care provider attitudes, lesbian, gay, and bisexual people cite the heterosexism of the health care setting as a major barrier to adequate care. Potential remedies for these problems will be discussed in Chapter 9.

EXERCISE: PREDICTORS OF NEGATIVE ATTITUDES

The following chart lists some of the factors that research has suggested predict or contribute to negative attitudes about lesbian, gay, and bisexual people (see Eliason, 1995, for a review of these studies). For each characteristic, circle the response that best fits your own situation:

Characteristics	Column 1	Column 2
Age	23-49	< 22 or > 49
Sex	female	male
Views on gender roles in society	nontraditional	traditional
Belong to a fundamentalist religion	no	yes
Attend church more than once per week	no	yes
Catholic or Protestant faith	no	yes
Not religious	yes	no
Republican	no	yes
Parents had/have negative views about homosexuality	no	yes
Conservative about all matters of sexuality	no	yes
Have a college education	yes	no
Have a friend or relative who is lesbian, gay, bisexual	yes	no
Grew up in the South or Midwest	no	yes
Believe that homosexuality is genetic/biological	yes	no
Sexual identity	gay, lesbian, bisexual	hererosexual, asesual

Now add up all your circled responses in Column 2. These are predictors of negative attitudes, not direct causes. The more predictors you have, the more likely it is that you grew up with or are currently exposed to homophobic attitudes. The purpose of this exercise is not to put blame on you, but to help you identify the roots of your attitudes. You cannot help, or change, your age, sex, where you grew up, or your parents' beliefs, but these historical and cultural factors have contributed to the person you are today and may influence your attitudes. This list can be used for self-analysis.

Sexual Identity and Developmental Transitions

ALTHOUGH HUMAN DEVELOPMENT IS A unique, dynamic, and complex process, most people experience some fairly predictable transitions that can help us predict and understand their behavior or attitudes at different ages. Chronological age markers are rough indicators of development, but we all use age as a convenient categorization scheme. I will do likewise and begin this discussion with childhood. Since sexual identity, as a conscious phenomenon, usually forms in adolescence or later, gender nonconforming behavior is a possible early sign of a lesbian, gay, or bisexual sexual identity. I will point out how difficult it is to discuss sexuality without also discussing sex and gender. In the later age groupings, sexual identity has a more direct influence on other life events and transitions.

CHILDHOOD

I knew I was queer when I was a small child. My voice was gentle and sweet. I avoided sports and all roughness. I played with the girls. I did not fit into the world around me. I knew the meaning of "heresy" before I entered kindergarten. Heresy was a boy who cried a lot when he got hurt. Heresy was a boy who couldn't throw a baseball. Heresy was a boy putting on girls' clothing. Heresy was me. As I got older, and fully entered the society of children, I met the key enforcer of social roles among children: the bully. The bully was the boy who defined me as queer to my peers. . . . I know a lot about bullies . . . they define the limits of acceptable conduct, appearance, and activities for children. They enforce rigid expectations. They are masters of

the art of humiliation and technicians of the science of terror-
ism. They wreaked havoc on my entire childhood. To this day,
their handprints, like a slap on the face, remain stark and de-
fined on my soul. When I was a young boy, the bully called me
names, stole my bicycle, and forced me off the playground. . . .
He made fun of me in front of the other children. . . . At different
times, I was subject to a wide range of degradation and
abuse . . . "de-pantsing," spit in the face, forced to eat play-
ground dirt. . . . The world of childhood was a cruel place for
me. (Eric Rofes, 1995, p. 79-80)

Since sex and gender are such powerful influences in our society, one
of the most noticeable ways that children can express difference is via
behavior that is considered inappropriate for their biological sex. Gender nonconformity is sometimes labeled as a psychiatric disorder (more
on this later); sometimes, it results in teasing and harassment from
peers; and often it causes discomfort in the adults around the nonconforming children, especially parents. Boys are much more likely to be
punished for gender nonconformity than girls. Historically, it has
seemed natural that some girls would envy the freedom that boys have
in their play activities and their advantages in the world; thus "tomboy"
behavior has been considered normal to a certain extent. Some girls
either persist in tomboy activities longer than other girls and become
suspect, or display these gender nonconforming attitudes to an extreme
(e.g., telling their parents that they wish to be boys). On the whole,
however, it's boys who are punished for gender nonconformity.

As noted earlier, some lesbian, gay, and bisexual people deviate
from the gender norms established by society. This link between gender and sexual identity has been studied from two vantage points.
First, researchers have asked lesbian, gay, or bisexual adults to recall
their childhood play activities and have determined whether these
were gender conforming or nonconforming behaviors. Second, children who have been diagnosed with a "gender identity disorder" have
been followed into adolescence or adulthood by researchers who look
for links between their childhood behaviors and their adult sexuality.

From the first vantage point, several studies have noted a high frequency of gender nonconforming childhood memories in lesbian, gay,
and bisexual people (Harry, 1982; Saghir & Robins, 1973; Whitam,
1977). A few recent studies will serve as examples. In Australia, Phillips

and Over (1992) studied male clients from four general medicine practices and one communicable disease clinic trying to avoid the bias in-
herent in using only members of gay organizations or clientele of gay
bars. The clients were given questionnaires in the clinic, and asked to
complete them at home and return them to the authors. Of the 139
clients who returned questionnaires, 54 were heterosexual men with an
average age of 28; 24, bisexual men with a mean age of 31; and 61, homosexual men with a mean age of 32. The three sexual identity groups
had similar levels of education, employment, and religious affiliation.
The men in the heterosexual and bisexual groups were mostly single,
with only 20% living in marriages or committed cohabitation. Of the gay
men, 11% were divorced or separated.

Respondents completed the Boyhood Gender Conformity Scale for
their childhood gender behaviors, and a Sex-Role Scale to measure current gender traits. There were no group differences on the Sex-Role
Scale, showing that the three groups had similar scores on current masculine and feminine traits. However, there were significant differences
between heterosexual and homosexual men on the childhood gender behaviors on 10 out of 20 items. Bisexual men differed from heterosexual
men on only two items (preference for boy's games and considered a
sissy). The bisexual men and gay men did not differ statistically on any
of the items. Using a stepwise discriminant analysis to identify items
that distinguished homosexual men from heterosexual men, the authors
identified seven key items that accurately classified 90% of the respondents. In order of their predictive power, these items were (1) engaged
in rough-and-tumble play, (2) imagined self as a sports figure, (3) imagined self as a dancer or model, (4) preference for boys' games, (5) desire
to grow up like father, (6) preference for girl's games, and (7) preference for the company of older women. Bisexual men had intermediate
scores, but they were closer to the gay men than the heterosexual men.
However, to rely only on mean scores is misleading, so Table 6.1 lists
four of the items and the percentage of men in each group who said
"yes" to that item. It is clear that not all gay or bisexual men were gender
nonconforming, and that some heterosexual men recalled some gender
nonconformity.

Phillip and Over (1995) also studied the childhood recollections of
heterosexual, bisexual, and lesbian women. The respondents likewise
were gathered from medical clinics and completed questionnaires. The
authors classified women by sexual identity in three ways. To simplify

TABLE 6.1. Gender Behaviors in Childhood Memories of Heterosexual, Bisexual, and Gay Adult Men

| | Percentage of "Yes" Answers | | |
Item	Heterosexual	Bisexual	Gay
Engaged in rough-and-tumble play	100%	88%	66%
Preference for boys' games	96	83	67
Preference for girls' games	17	50	67
Considered a sissy	0	17	28

Note. Adapted from Phillips and Over (1992).

this discussion, I will report the results using the most conservative definitions: A woman was classified as heterosexual if she gave a rating of 0 on the Kinsey scale and had experienced cross-sex but not same-sex orgasm since the age of 18. There were 78 heterosexuals by this definition. A woman was classified as a lesbian if she gave a rating of 6 on the Kinsey scale and had experienced same-sex but not cross-sex orgasm since the age of 18 ($n = 22$). The remainder of women ($n = 39$) were classified as bisexual. The results were similar to the men's study: There were no differences on the measure of current sex-role traits, but significant differences were associated with memories of childhood gender behaviors. Stepwise discriminant analyses showed that four items distinguished between heterosexual and lesbian women, correctly classifying 82% of heterosexuals and 73% of lesbians: (1) imagined self as a male character, (2) wished to become a mother, (3) preference for boys' games, and (4) considered a tomboy as a child. Like the bisexual men, bisexual women had intermediate scores, and the discriminant analysis was not as accurate when bisexuals were added—only 59% of the sample could be accurately classified. Table 6.2 shows some of the items on the scale and the percentage of women in each sexual identity group who reported these behaviors in childhood.

Being considered a tomboy was a common experience for all groups, and being a tomboy does not have the negative connotations that being a sissy has for boys. Because young girls are allowed a greater range of gender activities than boys, gender nonconformity is not as strongly linked to adult sexuality for women as it is for men.

Bailey, Miller, and Willerman (1993) studied 58 heterosexual men, 83 bisexual and homosexual men, 51 heterosexual women, 19 bisexual or lesbian women, and their mothers. The heterosexual respondents were

TABLE 6.2.   Gender Behaviors in Childhood Memories of Heterosexual, Bisexual, and Lesbian Adult Women

Item	Percentage of "Yes" Answers		
	Heterosexual	Bisexual	Lesbian
Imagined self as a male character	37%	62%	82%
Wished to become a mother	78	59	41
Preference for boys' games	63	79	86
Considered a tomboy	63	77	77

Note. Adapted from Phillips and Over (1995).

younger than the bisexual or homosexual respondents but were similar on other demographic characteristics. In this study, childhood was defined as before the age of 13, and mothers as well as their adult children were asked to rate childhood activities. Mothers' ratings for heterosexual and gay/bisexual sons differed on four items; gay/bisexual sons were rated as less masculine, nonathletic, more poorly adjusted, and less healthy. Mothers' ratings of heterosexual and lesbian/bisexual daughters also differed, with lesbian/bisexual daughters more often rated as masculine, less submissive, more poorly adjusted, less healthy, and more passive. Mothers' ratings of heterosexual daughters and sons revealed only one significant difference—sons were rated as more masculine.

Because the mothers' ratings of their adult children's behavior could be biased by their knowledge of the child's current sexual identity (as well as faulty memory and socially desirable responding), the lesbian, gay, and bisexual respondents were asked whether their mothers were aware of their sexual identities. Only two gay/bisexual men reported that their mothers definitely knew and another 23 thought that their mothers suspected. Nine lesbian/bisexual women said that their mothers knew and one thought she suspected. The theory was that if mothers' ratings reflected societal stereotypes about homosexuality, the ones who knew would have the most bias. There was no evidence to support this theory for males; however, for lesbian and bisexual women, maternal knowledge of their sexual identity was significantly related to their childhood ratings, perhaps reflecting the influence of negative societal stereotypes. In another interesting finding, there was no relationship between the respondents' self-ratings of childhood and their mothers' ratings. These findings suggest that the childhood memories alone, whether self-ratings or maternal ratings, are not an accurate predictor of adult sexual identity, as they are influenced by the retro-spective process—faulty memory, socially desirable responding, re-construction of the past to fit the current identity, and the powerful influence of societal stereotypes. It is also possible that lesbian, gay, and bisexual people who are the most "obvious" in their appearance, man-nerisms, or relationships as adults were more noticeably different as children. Their mothers may have recognized their difference early on, and suspect their child's adult sexual identity whether or not the child is aware of it.

To avoid the multitude of problems with self-report retrospective memories, some researchers have concentrated on prospective, longi-tudinal studies. These studies, which usually focus on a clinical sam-ple—generally boys who were brought to gender disorder clinics—can only be considered suggestive because they do not represent "normal" or random samples. Nevertheless, they shed light on the possible role of gender nonconformity as a precursor of male adult homosexual ori-entation. Less is known about the relationship between gender non-conformity in childhood in women and its effects on and relationship to adult sexual identity.

Zuger (1984) followed 55 boys who had been brought to a psychia-trist primarily because of parents' concern about "effeminate"[1] behav-ior. Some of these boys ($n = 6$) had already shown some homosexual behavior. On initial evaluation, they ranged from about 4 to 16 years of age. The gender nonconformity had begun very early for most sub-jects—47 of the 55 mothers noted differences by the time their sons had reached 6 years of age. The boys themselves reported that they had always felt different from other boys. The gender nonconforming be-havior that had distressed the mothers included feminine dressing (50%), aversion to boys' games (50%), stated desire to be female (43%), preference for girls as playmates (42%), playing with dolls (41%), and feminine gestures (40%). Follow-up interviews when the subjects were adolescents or young adults revealed the following pattern of sexual

---

[1]The term *effeminate* is widely used in many of the earlier studies of childhood, but it is also widely used in lay conversations about boys or men who have qualities often associated with women. The term has taken on a negative connotation, and there is no exact parallel for women. I prefer the more neutral term *gender nonconformity*, which does not perpetuate stereotypes.

identities: homosexual (64%), heterosexual (6%), uncertain (18%), and lost to follow-up (12%). If the lost to follow-up group is excluded, 73% were homosexual, 6% heterosexual, and 21% uncertain. However, among those designated by the author as homosexual were one homosexual transvestite and one homosexual transsexual.

This study has at least two major flaws that characterize many such studies—the lack of a normal comparison group and the subjective definition of sexual orientation. The author did not directly ask the young men about their sexuality—17 had self-disclosed and the rest were "diagnosed" as probable homosexuals by certain signs such as continued gender nonconformity, close association with known homosexuals, parents' opinions, or the opinions of other psychiatrists, all notoriously unreliable and indirect measures of homosexuality.

A better designed study was reported by Green (1985), who followed two groups of boys: 66 who were clinical referrals for gender nonconformity and 56 who were a matched sample of "normal" boys. The groups were matched on age, sex, sibling sequence, race, religion, parents' education, and parents' marital status. By race, 79% were European American, 8% were African American, 8% were Latinos, and 6% were of mixed races. The boys were initially evaluated when they were ages 3 to 11. Behaviors in childhood were assessed by parent questionnaires and semistructured interviews. Marked cross-gender behaviors characterized the clinical group, whereas the comparison group boys occasionally displayed some cross-gender behavior, but not to the extent or as frequently as the clinical group.

Although several families were lost to follow-up, 44 of the boys in the clinical sample and 34 of the comparison boys were evaluated in their adolescent years. Green determined their sexual identities using three methods; fantasy, actual sexual behavior, and penile response to pornographic pictures of males and females. For each measure, he assigned a Kinsey score (0 to 6), then averaged the scores from the different measures. The clinical group's sexual orientation scores ranged from 0 to 1, or heterosexual (32%), from 2 to 4, or bisexual (25%), and from 5 to 6, or homosexual (43%). The boys in the comparison group were all rated as heterosexual. In the clinical group of 44 boys, 12 had received extensive therapy, but the rates of homosexuality and bisexuality did not differ in the therapy and no-therapy groups.

Although most studies of childhood gender nonconformity are seriously flawed by retrospective data, nonrandom samples, and different methods of determining sexual identity, they suggest a link between gender nonconformity in childhood and adult sexual identity. In every study, a significant number of boys with gender nonconformity appear to develop a gay or bisexual identity as adults (and a smaller number become transgendered adults). What remains to be explained is why some gender nonconforming boys grow up to be heterosexual, and why some gender conforming children grow up to be lesbian, gay, or bisexual. Obviously, gender nonconformity alone is not the determining factor of sexual identity.

Many studies indicate that adult lesbian, gay, and bisexual people remember feeling different as children and often attribute this difference to gender nonconformity. Not until later—in adolescence or adulthood—do they identify it as a sexual difference. As our society changes, however, and children are exposed to more explicit sexuality (on TV, at the movies, in magazines and advertisements), they may begin to recognize sexual differences at earlier ages.

Should we intervene for gender nonconformity? Why do many adults seem so distressed when children exhibit cross-gender behaviors? Why do we have such strict gender roles anyway? The psychiatric diagnosis of "gender identity disorder" seems as outmoded today as the diagnosis of "homosexuality" was in earlier years. Children are diagnosed with gender identity disorders, not because they are inherently mentally ill, but because their behavior makes others uncomfortable. They suffer, not because of their behavior per se (their behavior may give them pleasure), but because of the societal stigma attached to cross-gender behavior (because of its perceived link to homosexuality). I believe that health care providers should be committed to removing gender identity disorder from the current edition of the *Diagnostic and Statistical Manual of Mental Disorders* (American Psychiatric Association, 1994), and to helping parents and teachers accept all children. Rigid gender roles contribute to and maintain sexism and heterosexism in our society. By considering gender as a continuum instead of as opposite male-female poles, we could allow a freer expression of human traits and would not need to force people into gender-defined roles.

When children exhibit gender nonconforming behaviors, we can accept them, encourage them to be themselves, and help them deal with teasing or harassment from peers. All children should be taught to respect difference and should understand that harassment is not acceptable; taunting gender nonconforming peers with verbal insults like "sissy," "fairy," and "fag" should earn firm punishment. Children who are gender nonconformers should not be punished by being taken to a psychiatrist for treatment of behavior that feels completely natural and normal to them. Taking these children for "help" gives a strong message that their parents think they are bad or sick, and can result in low self-esteem, shame, and guilt. Besides, studies show that treatment for gender nonconformity does not change adult sexual identity, or even current gender behaviors (Green, 1987).

ADOLESCENCE

> *I can't ever let anyone find out that I'm not straight. It would be so humiliating. My friends would hate me. They might even want to beat me up. And my family? I've overheard them. They've said they hate gays and even God hates gays, too. Gays are bad, and God sends bad people to hell. It really scares me when they talk that way because now they are talking about me [diary entry by 16-year-old Bobby Griffith, four years before he committed suicide]. (cited in Aarons, 1995, p. 57)*

The teen years are characterized by changes in the physical, cognitive, and emotional components of the individual. As the physical body literally erupts into adult sexual capabilities, the cognitive and emotional aspects often lag behind, creating a young person controlled by bodily urges and egocentrism. The adolescent years are marked by confusion about sexuality, and for most teens sexual experimentation. Peer pressures are stronger in adolescence than at any other time in life, adding to the turmoil. The media and the peer group send a strong message that teens should be sexual; parents, schools, and religions encourage them to "just say no." For teens who are sexually different, adolescence may be the hardest life transition they will face.

Bidwell (1988) described the "denied adolescence" of many lesbian, gay, and bisexual teens. Elements of the denied teen years include missing many of the rites of passage of dating, living with a terrible secret and the ever-present fear of discovery, a lack of positive role models leading to feelings of isolation, and a lack of trusted confidants. Bidwell noted, "The gradual discovery of who one is and how one relates to others requires extensive social interaction and experimentation. For most gay teens, this is simply impossible" (p. 5). As other teens begin to pair off in heterosexual dating couples and social groups, the lesbian, gay, or bisexual teen may begin to feel alienated: "At a time when heterosexual adolescents are learning to socialize, young gay people are learning how to hide" (Hetrick & Martin, 1984, p. 6).

Like the studies of childhood, most empirical research about sexual identity in adolescence relies on retrospective memories of lesbian, gay, and bisexual adults. These studies show that same-sex attractions generally occurred early in adolescence (12–14 for boys and 14–16 for girls; Saghir & Robins, 1973); same-sex sexual experiences typically followed a few years later, again with gay and bisexual men reporting earlier ages of same-sex sexual activity than lesbians or bisexual women.

There have been a few good prospective studies of adolescents—one of the most comprehensive studies was reported by Herdt and Boxer (1993), who studied 55 lesbian and bisexual young women and 147 gay and bisexual young men. Their data on sexual milestones suggested that sexual identity formation begins before puberty, as the age of first same-sex attractions was 10.1 for females and 9.6 for males (Table 6.3). Actual same-sex sexual experiences came during or after puberty, at an average age of 13 for boys and 15 for girls. A significant number of both boys (59%) and girls (80%) had other-sex sexual experiences as well—both at an average age of about 13.5. The patterns of first sexual experiences for lesbian and bisexual female teens were (1) same-sex, then other-sex, 34%; (2) other-sex, then same-sex, 45%; and (3) same-sex exclusively, 21%. For gay and bisexual male teens, the patterns were (1) same-sex, then other-sex, 36%; (2) other-sex, then same-sex, 22%; and (3) same-sex exclusively, 42%. Heterosexual experiences of these

TABLE 6.3. Sexual Milestones in Lesbian, Gay, and Bisexual Adolescents

Milestone	Mean Age of Occurrence	
	Boys ($n = 147$)	Girls ($n = 55$)
First same-sex attraction	9.6	10.1
First same-sex experience	13.1	15.2
First other-sex experience	13.7 ($n = 87$)	13.6 ($n = 44$)
Came out as lesbian, gay, or bisexual	16.0	16.0

Note. Adapted from Herdt & Boxer (1993).

teens were attributed to desperately wanting to be heterosexual (passing), curiosity, peer pressure and, for females, coercion by the men they dated. The high number of lesbian, gay, and bisexual teens with heterosexual experiences points out the need to consider pregnancy, date rape, and similar issues as potential problems of all teens, not only heterosexuals.

Internalized homophobia is a major risk factor for lesbian, gay, and bisexual teens (Shidlo, 1994). This self-hatred stemming from a belief in negative stereotypes may take months or even years to overcome before they can develop a realistic and positive view of themselves and other lesbian, gay, and bisexual people. In addition to self-hatred, internalized homophobia in adolescents may result in efforts to pass as heterosexual, depression, unsafe sex (heterosexual as well as same-sex), and substance abuse. Overcoming internalized homophobia is a resocialization process (Herdt & Boxer, 1993) that involves unlearning stereotypes, learning facts, accepting self and others as unique, acknowledging the diversity of lesbian, gay, and bisexual communities, dating and finding community, and recognizing the oppressive effects of homophobia on daily life (i.e., putting their problems into the larger political framework rather than blaming themselves for their parents' rejection or other homophobic reactions). These teens may also need to give up previously internalized heterosexual life goals and set new ones. The loss of previous goals may involve some degree of grieving. This is even more true for parents of lesbian, gay, and bisexual teens—they may have to drastically revise the life goals they had fantasized for their children.

The major reproductive transition for adolescent females is the onset of menstruation and capability for childbearing. There appears to be no research concerning lesbian or bisexual women's responses to or adjustment to menstruation. It could be hypothesized that the subset of lesbians who reject or fear heterosexual femininity might react badly to the onset of menstruation. Anecdotally, I know a woman who believed for all of her childhood that she would eventually become a man. When she began to menstruate at age 13, she went into a year-long depression. It took her another five or six years to recognize that she didn't really want to be a man; that she wanted to love women and have the same privileges that men in our society have. However, lesbians vary so widely in their degree of "femininity" and attitudes about being women that no generalizations can be made about potential reactions to menstruation. The factors that predict healthy adaptation to menstruation in heterosexual teens—mothers' attitudes about menstruation and amount of preparation for the event—most likely also predict adaptation for lesbian teens.

Gay and bisexual male teens in puberty may begin to face even more harassment from their male peers than they did in childhood. Locker rooms and gym classes can be particularly stressful and humiliating, especially for the nonathletic young man. Over half of lesbian, gay, and bisexual teens report having been harassed, threatened, or beaten by their classmates because of their known or perceived sexual identities (Savin-Williams, 1994).

The main problems of lesbian, gay, or bisexual adolescents stem from two interrelated factors—the social stigma of homosexuality and bisexuality and the lack of adequate sex education. These factors combine to make adolescence a lonely, isolated time for many, and a potentially dangerous period as well. Sexual experimentation has always carried many risks for teens, not least of which are pregnancy and sexually transmitted infections. With the advent of HIV, however, lack of knowledge about sex has become deadly. The following sections describe problems that can arise from negative societal attitudes coupled with inadequate sex education.

Coming Out

Coming out to family and friends is stressful at any age, but for the teen, it poses even greater risks than for the adult. Many families react negatively, and unlike the adult, the adolescent cannot just walk away. Most lesbian, gay, and bisexual people carefully consider the issue for months, even years, before coming out to parents. Yet many parents dismiss the disclosure as a fad or a phase that the teen will outgrow, trivializing the teen's tremendous courage in revealing her/himself. Other parents tell children they are mentally or morally ill and take them to a psychiatrist, or arrange for religious counseling. Yet other parents respond with violence and/or reject their own children. For the financially and emotionally dependent teen, this loss of support can be devastating and may lead to homelessness.

Theoretically, coming out to self and others appears to be a step toward healthy adjustment to sexual identity, but it is complicated for many teens. Besides fearing violence or rejection from parents, lesbian, gay, and bisexual teens of color may rely on their families for support of their racial difference, and fear that coming out would mean loss of entire supportive communities (Weston, 1991). Lesbian, gay, and bisexual teens from families with conservative religious beliefs or "traditional values" may also be less likely to come out to family (Newman & Muzzonigro, 1993).

Until there are major changes in society, coming out to parents will remain a risky business for teens. Many lesbian, gay, and bisexual people wait until they are economically independent and have developed a strong support system before coming out to family. Ironically, parental acceptance is the factor that best predicts whether lesbian, gay, and bisexual teens will feel comfortable with their own sexual identity (Savin-Williams, 1989). This fact points out the need for greater education of the general public, so that families are not totally unprepared for the coming out of a family member.

Depression and Suicide

Several recent studies have found the risks for suicide to be much higher among lesbian, gay, and bisexual teens because of internalized homophobia and social stigmatization. A U.S. government report found that over 30% of all teen suicides are related to concern about sexual identity (Gibson, 1994). Among lesbian and bisexual female teens, suicidal thoughts and attempts are reported by a significant number and possibly in greater frequency than in gay male teens (Remafedi, 1994). Rates of suicide attempts in the general population of adolescents are 8%–13%, but in lesbian, gay, and bisexual teens, the rates are 25%–42% (Hershberger & D'Augelli, 1995). Suicide attempts in lesbian, gay, and bisexual teens are often linked to sexual milestones, such as self-definition as being gay or coming out to a friend or family member (Remafedi, Farrow, & Deisher, 1991). Suicide is a complex and difficult phenomenon, and for lesbian, gay, and bisexual teens appears to be the result of an interaction of their own acceptance of their homo- or bisexuality, the amount of family support they receive, and other family variables unrelated to their sexuality.

Violence, Homelessness, and Prostitution

"Gay-bashing," or physical violence directed at people solely because of their perceived sexual identity, is on the rise and is most often perpetrated by 14–19-year-old males—the classmates of the lesbian, gay, and bisexual teen (Herek & Berrill, 1992). Additionally, many teens who reveal their sexual identity suffer violence from their families (Berrill, 1992). Less extreme, but just as damaging, is the potential for rejection by family and peers. Recent data on homeless teens suggest that perhaps 30%–40% of them are lesbian, gay, or bisexual teens who have been kicked out of their homes by their families, or who feared rejection and/or violence from their families (Savin-Williams, 1994). Many of these homeless teens are also HIV positive. Survival on the streets rests on only a few options, primarily prostitution and drug dealing. Male prostitutes often report very low self-esteem and a desire to quit hustling, but they do not think they have any other options. Ironically, the lesbian, gay, or bisexual teens who ran away from home to escape abusive parents or parents with substance abuse are even more vulnerable to these same ills on the streets.

Sexually Transmitted Infections, HIV, and Pregnancy

In 1994, 417 new cases of AIDS were reported to the Center for Disease Control (CDC) in 13–19-year-olds, and 13,198 cases in 20–29-year-olds (most of whom were infected during their adolescent years (Centers for Disease Control Newsletter (CDC), February 3, 1995; see Stine, 1995). Adolescents are vulnerable to all types of sexually transmitted infections (STIs) and to pregnancy for a number of reasons. First, they often lack information—schools are reluctant to teach explicit sex education for fear of community reprisal and parents are unprepared to teach this material at home. Even if they have information, adolescents are vulnerable because of the developmental characteristics of the stage; they often have a sense of invulnerability, are risk takers, are experimenting with sexuality, and rebel against authority. If they do have an STI or suspect a pregnancy, they might not recognize the symptoms, or not know where to get help.

Lesbian and bisexual female teens have to deal with both homophobia and sexism, and may be pressured to be heterosexually active more intensely than gay male youth. Risks for pregnancy and STIs are relatively high. Gay and bisexual male teens may not use or have adequate knowledge about contraception and engage in unprotected heterosexual sex to "prove their masculinity."

Guidelines for Working with Lesbian, Gay, and Bisexual Teens

The following suggestions come primarily from Remafedi (1985) and Bidwell (1988). Health care providers who work with adolescents know how difficult this population can be. Many teens are suspicious of authority figures and unlikely to disclose any personal information. Lesbian, gay, and bisexual teens may be even more wary of health care providers who they fear will talk to their parents. Keeping this natural reticence of the adolescent in mind, health care providers can consider the following:

1. If the teen comes out, avoid empty reassurances, anecdotal information, or personal bias. If you cannot discuss sexuality issues objectively, refer the teen to someone who can.

2. If a teen announces concern or confusion about her/his sexual identity, do not attempt to apply a label. Instead, provide accurate information and present heterosexuality, homosexuality, and bisexuality as equally valid options. Assist teens in achieving a sexual identity on their own.

3. Assure the teen that your discussion will be confidential, and then make sure that it is.

4. Be prepared for family discord and anticipate potential problems. Help the teen to develop a plan for coming out to family if she/he has not yet done so. Offer to role-play the coming out speech with the teen and try out a number of different parental reactions.

5. Every adolescent client needs a thorough sexual history and a discussion of sexual matters such as contraception, safer sex, and resources available in your community.

6. If you are unsure of the teen's sexual identity, you can provide openings for her/him to disclose or ask questions. Bidwell (1988) suggested a question such as "A lot of young men (or women) your age are worried about feeling attracted to others of their own sex. Have you ever had these feelings or worried about them?" (p. 6). Don't wait for disclosure, because many teens fear rejection or disapproval from you and probably will not disclose voluntarily.

7. Know your local resources for lesbian, gay, and bisexual teens. Are there teen support groups at the schools, mental health clinics, or elsewhere? Is there a hotline or a center? Which adolescent counselors are supportive? Are there other positive role models in the community? Does the library have books or videos about sexual identity for teens?

8. Be aware of potential psychosocial problems, especially depression, suicide, and substance abuse. Refer as needed to those supportive counselors.

Working with Parents of Lesbian, Gay, and Bisexual Teens

Many health care providers will also work with parents, who may or may not know or suspect their teen's sexual identity. The coming out process may be a time of crisis for the family, and health care providers can ease the transition by:

1. Modeling acceptance of the teen and helping parents work through the initial shock.

2. Providing accurate, up-to-date information to combat myths and stereotypes.

3. Helping parents to understand that counseling (religious or psychological) is not effective since homosexuality and bisexuality are not mental or psychological disorders. Trying to take their children to a counselor sends a message that the parents think they are sick. On the other hand, the parents may benefit from counseling to help them adjust to the news and be more supportive of their child.

4. Referring them to a parent support group, such as Parents and Friends of Lesbians and Gays (PFLAG), or if unavailable in your community, other parents who have survived the coming out process.

Health care providers need to be committed to providing better care for adolescents. In fact, one health care organization announced:

The American Academy of Pediatrics reaffirms the physician's responsibility to provide comprehensive health care and guidance for all adolescents, including gay and lesbian adolescents and those young people struggling with issues of sexual orientation. The deadly consequences of AIDS and adolescent suicide underscore the critical need to address and seek to prevent the major physical and mental health problems that confront gay and lesbian youths in their transition to a healthy adulthood. (Committee on Adolescence, 1993, p. 633)

Young Adulthood

As I grew up through my teens, I never had any relationship with a woman, and I don't think anybody ever treated me different. I had a family, I had a tennis life, I had a boyfriend. . . . I never thought there was anything strange about being gay. Other people would make jokes, but I couldn't figure out why these people were "sick." I knew it was more tolerated in the West than in Czechoslovakia. There, they would put you in the sanatorium for crazy people, literally. . . . It was just a matter of time for me. I had to get other parts of my life in order first. . . . When it finally happened, it was with somebody older than me, a woman I met in the States and it seemed so natural. . . . When it finally happened, I said, This is easy and right. . . . I wanted privacy but I was also uncomfortable about pretending to be something I wasn't. Somebody once said to me, "Society isn't ready for it." And I told her, "Hey, we're society, too." (Martina Navratilova, 1993, pp. 24–25)

Psychologists have described the developmental transitions of young adults as including establishment of intimate relationships, seeking out committed partners and beginning a family, achieving full independence from families of origin, and exploring and establishing a career or job. Much of the early research focused on young adult women and the development of relationships and family, and young adult men and the development of independence and careers. As gender roles change slowly in our society, women and men are equally likely to experience transitions related to career and family. Being lesbian, gay, or bisexual can alter the experiences of all these developmental transitions. Before discussing these "normal" young adult transitions, I will review the coming out process briefly.

Coming Out

Most lesbian, gay, and bisexual people come out in their young adult years, and many have their first acknowledged same-sex relationship at this time. Most were aware of their sexuality much earlier, however, and may have come out to themselves in adolescence. Moving away from home allows them the freedom to explore a lesbian, gay, or bisexual identity more fully and they generally begin to disclose this information to others. There is quite a large body of research on the college undergraduate, because of their availability to researchers. Much less is known about working class or non-college-educated lesbian, gay, and bisexual people at any age.

Rhoads (1995) conducted interviews with 40 gay male students about their coming out experiences and found four general themes. The respondents viewed coming out as a continual process of change via a dramatic increase in self-awareness and self-confidence. For many, coming out led to a heightened awareness of political issues revolving around gay rights. Respondents also reported negative consequences of coming out, such as family disruptions, loss of friends, and ongoing experiences of harassment and discrimination. Residence halls were a notable location for harassment, but many also noted that issues of sexual identity were absent, marginalized, or vilified in their classrooms. One student noted, "I don't feel very safe on campus . . . you just never know when a group of frat boys or jock types . . . you know those who are probably most closeted—are going to beat your face in because you remind them of what they can't admit to" (Rhoads, 1995, p. 71).

Goff (1990) described the same phenomenon—sexual confusion among some college males (and presumably other young adult men as well). He suggested that male socialization for intimacy is typically rather poor so that some young men have difficulty forming intimate relationships with women. They then worry that they are sexually abnormal, maybe gay, and because these feelings are totally unacceptable, the young man reacts with denial, substance abuse, and/or reaction formation. The reaction formation is a defense mechanism to protect the man from his own feelings by expressing homophobia outwardly. Thus, some of the most virulently homophobic men are, ironically, masking their own sexual confusions and fears of being gay.

Forming Intimate Relationships

As Bidwell (1988) noted, lesbian, gay, and bisexual people who were denied their adolescent dating rites may exhibit some characteristics of adolescence when they launch romantic relationships in young adulthood. Erik Erikson proposed that identity must be firmly established before an individual is capable of an intimate relationship: For the lesbian, gay, or bisexual person, the age of coming out becomes the marker for the beginning of identity formation. Until a person feels comfortable with the identity and achieves some level of self-acceptance, intimate relationships will be difficult. Compared with their heterosexual peers who may have had 10 or more years of dating experience prior to the first committed relationship, the lesbian, gay, or bisexual young adult may still be learning dating etiquette—especially since the heterosexual rules do not apply to same-sex dating.

Klinkenberg and Rose (1994) studied dating scripts of lesbians and gay men. Scripts are highly organized plans that guide our behavior. For heterosexuals, well-defined dating scripts follow gender role divisions in society—they designate men as initiating the date, choosing the activity, and initiating sexual activity. Women are scripted to accept or not accept the date, and to control whether or not sexual activity occurs. There are no set scripts for same-sex dating, leading to more confusion, but also to more potential for flexibility. In this study, 51 gay men and 44 lesbians completed surveys about dating (they were 88% White, 4% African American, 3% Native American, 3% Latino, and 1% Asian American).

Lesbians' and gay men's dating scripts for first dates had many similarities, but the gay men's scripts were more likely to include sexual activity and alcohol use. More men expected sex on a first date (22%) than women (15%). Lesbians' scripts more often contained mention of intimacy and emotional expression. Safer sex was not a usual part of dating scripts; only four men and no women mentioned it. Unlike heterosexual dating scripts, the gay and lesbian dating scripts included calling the date immediately after the date ended and discussion of topics such as coming out. Otherwise, the dating scripts were quite similar for same-sex and other-sex dating.

Mays, Cochran, and Rhue (1993) conducted interviews with eight African American lesbians in relationships with other African American women. As a group, they were more likely to have experienced discrimination because of race and gender than because of sexuality, but most of them were not out at work. In their African American communities, none of them were experiencing negative effects because of their relationships, but partners were introduced as "friends" and were not openly discussed. Some of the women had been in relationships with European American women in the past, and had reported feeling less welcome at family and community events. One woman noted that although she and her partner were of the same race, racism negatively impacted their relationship as they argued constantly about skin color and beauty standards. Some women shunned the lesbian community because of encountering racism there, and because of being isolated in the African American community they often had difficulty finding partners and building support systems. Many African American lesbians have children and relatively more heterosexual experience than do European American lesbians, further complicating their relationships. Relationships can be tainted or strengthened by racism, internalized racism, sexism, and homophobia.

Commitment to a Partner and Beginning a Family

Our society is family-oriented, and we are all socialized to want the ideal family; lesbian, gay, and bisexual people are no different. Same-sex families, however, receive no or very limited validation from the institutions of society such as religion, law, education, and the media. Individual health care providers can provide this validation by accepting these families. Lesbian, gay, and bisexual adults who have children from previous relationships, and are forming new relationships, are much like blended, or stepfamilies among heterosexuals—they will have many of the same problems. For additional information, review Chapter 4, which focused on family issues for lesbian, gay, and bisexual people.

Career and Work Issues

Young adulthood is a time of career exploration. Heterosexual young adults can be open and honest about their relationships in job interviews and at the workplace. Lesbian, gay, and bisexual people risk loss of job and harassment and discrimination from coworkers if they come out. Many college students face the agonizing choice of going back into the closet for employment purposes after the relative freedom of college, or limiting their employment options by being out in job interviews. Do they choose a conservative career with the potential for a good income and opportunity for advancement if it means returning to the closet? Do they put membership in gay organizations, where they may have had leadership roles, on their résumés? Will their job options be restricted by geography—such as selecting large urban areas with lesbian, gay, and bisexual communities rather than taking a great job in a smaller, more rural environment? Lee Badgett (1996) found that the decision to disclose sexual identity at work is complex, but that lesbian, gay, and bisexual people would much rather be honest with their coworkers and bosses—hiding significant relationships is extremely difficult and entails considerable loss of personal integrity. Thus, many lesbian, gay, and bisexual people are "downwardly mobile"; they select jobs in human service agencies or other "liberal" environments, are self-employed, or accept positions that do not match their educational qualifications.

MIDDLE ADULTHOOD

I see the beautiful, soft, voluptuous body and face of a grown woman of almost 50 long and richly satisfying years of growing. . . . I'm as fascinated with the ways the outside of me is changing as I am with the ways the inside of me is changing. I am growing paradoxically older and younger at one and the same time. I've become so much more gentle with myself emotionally and psychologically as I've felt freer, without criticism or judgment, to become conscious of my inner limits and frailties. . . . With each day and year, I am more and more willing to allow myself to be just exactly however I am. (Robyn Posin, 1991, p. 145)

Developmental theorists point to midlife as a time of potential crisis or major life transition; a period of questioning one's life choices and deciding whether or not to make changes in careers, relationships, or priorities. Some theorists have suggested that there are two underlying crises in midlife—accepting one's own mortality and achieving a sense of generativity (leaving something behind for future generations). In the older theories, the midlife crisis for men often centered on perceived loss of youth and questions of career choices. For women, the biological change of life, menopause, and the launching of children into adulthood (empty nest syndrome) were thought to lead to midlife crisis. As gender roles have grown more flexible, however, the psychological aspects of midlife have become more similar for heterosexual women and men. How might lesbian, gay, and bisexual people experience midlife differently than heterosexuals? First, a word of caution. As Kimmel and Sang (1995) pointed out, we must couch our discussions within the particular historical context of the people we are discussing. Lesbian, gay, and bisexual people who are middle-aged today may have come out prior to the gay liberation movements; many have been leaders or were heavily involved in those movements; and they were in early midlife already when the AIDS epidemic began. In their adolescence and young adult years, they were more likely to have been isolated and felt a greater need to hide their sexuality than do young people today. They had fewer visible role models and less access to information about sexuality. Future generations will have had different experiences that affect their developmental transitions through the life course.

Many people have written about the double standard in aging for heterosexual women and men. Heterosexual women, who depend heavily on physical appearance for their sense of worth, tend to be more afraid of aging than men, who are valued for their accomplishments. The advertising in women's magazines fuels this fear by urging women to do something about their wrinkles, gray hair, or sagging breasts. The greatest compliment for an older woman is for others to think she is younger than she is. Some authors have suggested that a double standard also exists for lesbian, gay, and bisexual people, but that it is gay men who are more afraid of aging. Many lesbian and bisexual women have rejected the traditional beauty standards for women and are not as much affected by societal standards. Lesbian culture may even value gray hair and wrinkles and focus more on the inner person than the outer body. Gay and bisexual male culture, however, has been much more attuned to standards of male beauty—tight, toned muscles and a youthful appearance. Thus, gay and bisexual men and heterosexual women may share this concern about changing physical appearance and aging as they attempt to attract and retain the attention of men (Siever, 1994). Friend (1987) described the potential for "accelerated aging" in gay and bisexual men, or the subjective feeling of being old at a younger age than expected. This theory suggests that while heterosexual men generally are at their peak in midlife, many middle-aged gay and bisexual men feel old in their youth-oriented culture.

Reproductive Transitions: Menopause

The major reproductive transition in midlife for women is menopause, or the cessation of childbearing capacity. Related to the physical changes of midlife, many researchers have proposed that there are emotional consequences to the loss of childbearing capacity and to the "empty nest syndrome," which require a shift in identities from mother and caregiver to other roles (Troll, 1989). Lesbians with children may need to deal with the same issues, but lesbians who have chosen not to reproduce or raise children may have very different responses. Many of these women may view menopause as a freeing experience—a liberation from pads and tampons and monthly annoyances (Neugarten, Wood, Kraines, & Loomis, 1963). Since lesbians as a group (not necessarily as individuals) are less invested in traditional feminine ideals, the physical changes of midlife such as facial hair, graying hair, wrinkles, and a more androgynous appearance may carry fewer potential consequences.

One way that lesbians, as a group, differ from heterosexual women, is that they are more likely to live alone at midlife. Bradford and Ryan (1991) found that 51% of the middle-aged lesbians in their sample lived with a partner, whereas 69% of heterosexual women lived with spouses. As a consequence, financial worries were five times more prevalent in the lesbian sample, and 27% had no health insurance. Although the researchers found no differences in the general health of midlife lesbians and women in general, lesbians as a group were less likely to have access to quality health care if they became ill. These financial worries may seem surprising; presumably, lesbians are more likely to have been continuously employed and career oriented than heterosexual women, and thus should have more financial security. As previously noted, however, they may not have pursued careers or jobs commensurate with their qualifications; women face both the "glass ceiling" and fears of discovery of their sexual identities.

Midlife "crises" for lesbian and bisexual women, much like those of men, involve striving for balance between work and relationships. Many describe the need for more time with their partners and complain of spending too much of their time together talking about work. Sang (1991) found that although most lesbians liked their jobs, they wished to be less work-oriented in the future. She also found that 76%

of the lesbians in her sample felt that midlife was the best time of their lives; another study found that midlife lesbians felt more confident, had more perspective, were better able to resolve conflicts, and felt wiser than they had in young adulthood (Fertitta, 1987).

Another potential issue for some women at midlife is coming out as a lesbian. A substantial body of literature shows that sexual identity change can occur at any time in the lifespan, and that many women embrace a lesbian identity relatively late in life (e.g., Charbonneau & Lander, 1991). The coming out process may be very different for the middle-aged woman than for the adolescent. It may necessitate major life changes—a divorce or living independently for the first time, coming out to children, finding a new community of friends and lovers and giving up the old. The reasons for coming out in midlife may also be different—coming out at an older age may be due to becoming politicized by the women's movement, not being able to deal with men anymore, a feeling that there is a greater likelihood of achieving intimacy with a woman than a man, or just happening to fall in love with a woman for the first time.

Some studies suggest that there are changes in sexuality with midlife—that some women report a decreased frequency and interest in sex. Only a few studies have examined lesbian midlife and sexuality. Cole and Rothblum (1991) studied 41 lesbians aged 43-68 (mean age of 52). All were currently sexually active, and 56% were in committed relationships of an average length of 7.3 years (range, 8 months-27 years). Most reported that the frequency of sex had not changed since menopause (46%), whereas 27% said the frequency had decreased and 15% said sexual activity had increased. Kirkpatrick (1989) suggested that sexual activity may change in midlife: Genital contact may decrease in frequency, but expression of feelings, physical touch, and intimacy may increase. She reported that lesbian couples in midlife generally report greater satisfaction with their sex lives than couples of other ages or other sexual identities.

Men at Midlife

There has been even less research about gay and bisexual men at midlife than about lesbian and bisexual women. However, there are some suggestions of the ways that gay and bisexual men might differ from heterosexual men, thus altering their midlife experiences. First, gay and bisexual men may experience a glass ceiling if they are out at work or are perceived to be gay or bisexual, making work more stressful. On the other hand, gay and bisexual men who do not have children may invest more time and effort into their careers, making them even more work-oriented than some heterosexual men. Blumstein and Schwartz (1983) found some evidence to the contrary. They found that 51% of the gay men in their sample (average age, 35), were predominantly relationship-focused while only 16% were predominantly work-focused. Relationship satisfaction was highest if both partners were relationship-focused, but most couples consisted of one relationship-focused partner and one work-focused partner.

Middle-aged gay and bisexual men may show less change in sexuality than lesbians, as male socialization in our society is more sex oriented than female socialization. Gay and bisexual men may decrease the frequency of sex somewhat from young adulthood to midlife, but generally they maintain a relatively high frequency and satisfaction of sexual activity (Kimmel & Sang, 1995).

Older Adulthood

Shevy Healy (1994), a 70-year-old retired clinical psychologist, had this to say about older lesbians:

> I would like to generalize a bit about what I see as special, unique, and significant about us as a group. . . . We are not docile. We do not accept the orthodoxies that women are here to serve and rely on men, are subservient to men, are not as valuable or as important as men. We are specifically nonconformist in that regard since each one of us, either from the start or later in life (sometimes quite late), has broken from the mold of mainstream heterosexual relationships. . . . We do not identify ourselves, nor do we want others to identify us as the "grandmothers" of the world, although many of us may, in fact, have grandchildren. We have a broader vision of our lives. On the other hand, we do now and have in the past placed a high premium on our own independence and self-reliance. . . . This also means that in our old age we may have considerable resistance to giving up any of our hard-won independence. . . . Others of us whose lesbianism came to the attention of their families early

*on experienced unspeakable horrors, from forced institutional-
ization in mental hospitals to hysterectomies and lobotomies.
There are those of us who have been ostracized by family and
friends, fired from jobs, dishonorably discharged from the service, scorned and ridiculed. . . . But our oppressions, while ex-
acting their price, have also taught us to be resourceful and to
develop special and sophisticated coping strategies that have en-
abled us to survive. (pp. 110-112)*

Older lesbian, gay, and bisexual people are invisible both in mainstream society, and in lesbian, gay, and bisexual organizations and communities. Little research has been directed to the issue of aging sexual
minorities. Older lesbian, gay, and bisexual people have to face the combined effects of ageism and heterosexism (as well as sexism, racism, and
classism for many), after having lived through much more repressive
times. Ageist stereotypes insist that older people are "asexual," thus few
consider that the older adult could be lesbian, gay, or bisexual.

One of the first studies of older gay men was conducted by Ray Berger
(1980). He surveyed 112 gay men who were age 40 and older (41-77).
They were all White and most were well-educated. Overall, he found a
high level of self-acceptance and life satisfaction with low levels of depression and anxiety about homosexuality. Most of the sample were still
sexually active (only 6% had no sex in the previous 6 months, compared
with 61% who had sex at least weekly). The men who were involved in
the gay community tended to show the greatest psychological adjustment, and the ones in a relationship were most satisfied with their lives.
Older respondents were generally better adjusted than the younger respondents, lending some credence to the "midlife crisis" theory.

More recent studies have highlighted some potential areas of concern for older lesbian, gay, and bisexual adults, such as living arrangements, involvement in the gay community, and health care needs.

Deevy (1990) noted that the nursing literature is beginning to acknowledge the existence of lesbian clients, but that nursing in general
still has a heterosexist bias. The first article concerning homosexuality
to appear in the gerontological literature was in 1982 (Noyes, 1982) and
did not mention lesbians. Deevy has tried to correct this oversight by
conducting a survey of 78 lesbians who were over the age of 50 (34 were
age 60 or older). Eighty percent were college educated and they reported a wide range of occupations such as teaching, nursing, farming,

banking, and chemist. Previous heterosexual marriages were reported by 42% and 31% had children. The majority had a positive attitude about aging (80%), and most were sexually active (50% lived with a lover). The age at which they had come out as lesbians covered an incredible range: 23% came out in their teens, 33% came out in their 20s, 14% came out in their 30s, 15% came out in their 40s, 12% in their 50s, and two came out when they were in their 60s! Because of growing up in much more restrictive times than now, many had bad experiences coming out, and 10% were out to no one. Fifty-four percent reported that they had feared discovery, and 31% had faced family disapproval. Deevy noted that older lesbian women have a number of potential health concerns; they do infrequent breast self-exams, have a somewhat higher alcohol consumption rate, are more likely to be overweight, and have a skepticism about health care systems that may delay health care seeking.

Adelman (1990) compared 27 gay men with 25 lesbians whose average age was in the mid-60s. All were White and from San Francisco. Most of them lived alone (32), and although 42 were retired, 10 still worked full time (4 men and 6 women), and 14 worked part time (6 men and 8 women). Women may need to work longer than men, since women earn less and are more likely to have jobs without retirement benefits. Adelman found that a significant minority of the sample had not disclosed their sexuality to anyone at work (26%) or to relatives (14%). The group was fairly evenly split by their involvement in the gay community; 21 had low involvement and 26 had high involvement. When she conducted a discriminant analysis to predict adjustment to aging, she found good adjustment was related to satisfaction with being gay, low self-criticism, few psychosomatic problems, and to having experimented as a gay person before self-definition as gay. Predictors of high life satisfaction included considering homosexuality as an important part of life, low disclosure at work, low involvement with other gay people, early age of awareness of homosexual feelings, and a decrease in the importance of homosexuality in later years. Adelman suggested that older lesbian and gay adults may have learned to manage the stigma of homosexuality by "compartmentalization" stemming from early socialization experiences that involved hiding their sexuality from others and leading double lives. Low involvement with gay friends or organizations that results from this perceived need for secrecy is a form of coping that may decrease in future generations.

Quam and Whitford (1992) studied 39 lesbian and 41 gay male adults over the age of 50 (50-73). More women lived with a partner (70%) than men (40%), but more women were in poor health (13%) than men (5%). More lesbians had annual incomes of less than $20,000 (41%) than men (27%). There were also differences in their social lives. Older gay men were more likely to go to gay bars (48% had gone to one in the past year compared with 23% of the lesbians), whereas lesbians were more likely to attend lesbian, gay, and bisexual social groups (77% compared with 53% of men). Quam and Whitford found that participation in community social events was positively related to satisfaction with the aging process and good health. The major concerns of this group included discrimination due to sexuality (50%), finances (26% of the women; 2% of the men), and health problems (21% of the women; 5% of the men). A significant number thought that being lesbian or gay helps in the aging process (68%) because of an accepting and supportive community, because the stress of being different leads to better coping skills, and because sexual identity status forces people to plan ahead for aging. Only 18% thought that being gay hindered the aging process, citing increased feelings of loneliness, difficulty forming long-lasting relationships, and fear of discrimination from health care systems as major concerns. None of these respondents were involved in gay community events. Eighteen percent thought that being gay neither helped nor hindered aging. A multiple regression analysis found that four variables predicted saying that being gay helped the aging process: acceptance of aging, younger age, living with someone, and absence of loneliness. The variables that predicted saying that being gay hinders aging were lack of acceptance of aging and older age. The authors concluded that the main concerns of older lesbian and gay adults were largely the same as those of older heterosexuals—loneliness, health, and finances—but were compounded by the stigma of homosexuality.

Elder Services and Lesbian, Gay, and Bisexual People

Behney (1995) surveyed 24 agencies on aging and 121 lesbians and gay men over the age of 60 (63 female and 58 male) about aging services. The agencies reported that most had no services specifically designed for or targeted to lesbian, gay, and bisexual people (96%). Only 17% had any staff training about homosexuality, but 88% said they were willing to undergo such training if it were available. Most of the agencies (79%) had never had any contact or communication with area lesbian, gay, or bisexual organizations, and 46% thought that lesbian, gay, and bisexual elders would not be welcome at senior centers if their sexual identities were known.

The lesbian, gay, and bisexual elders were mostly open about their sexuality (84%) and content with their sexuality (74%). Most (72%) were hesitant to use elder services because they did not trust the staff. Some (19%) had been involved with a senior center, and 62% thought that there should be separate services for lesbian, gay, and bisexual clients (compared with 64% of the agencies who thought that there should not be separate services).

Some larger cities are developing separate programs and outreach strategies for lesbian, gay, and bisexual elders. Table 6.4 lists some resources for gerontological or geriatric practitioners. In 1995, the White House Conference on Aging ("WHCoA") addressed sexuality issues for the first time and drafted a resolution entitled "Protecting the Rights of Older Citizens and Legal Residents against Discrimination," which included protection by race, age, and sexual orientation (see "WHCoA helps coalesce policy agenda," 1995). The recommendations included:

TABLE 6.4. Information Sources for Lesbian, Gay, and Bisexual Elder Services

Joe Brabant, Editor
SageNet
Box 2102, Suite D
Ottawa, ON, Canada
(613) 746-7279

Arlene Kochman, Executive Director
Sage
305 Seventh Avenue
New York, NY 10001
(212) 741-2247

Marcia Freedman
Lesbian & Gay Aging Issues Network (LGAIN)
American Society on Aging
833 Market Street, Suite 511
San Francisco, CA 94103-1824
(415) 974-9615

- Ensuring access to aging services (primarily by better education of staff).
- Developing health care prevention and education policies addressing risk factors for gay/lesbian elders.
- Addressing homophobia and eliminating the presumption of heterosexuality among providers and researchers.
- Eliminating legal and social barriers facing caregivers and survivors.
- Ensuring that fair housing practices include gay and lesbian elders in and remove barriers to development of sensitive housing alternatives.

EXERCISE: PLANNING FOR OUR OLD AGE

Whatever age you are now, imagine what you might be like and what you might be doing 20 years from now. How are you planning for your future? What do you think you will worry about the most? If you are heterosexual, imagine how your future planning might differ if you were lesbian, gay, or bisexual. If you are lesbian, gay, or bisexual, what are you doing to plan for your future?

CHAPTER SEVEN

Lesbian and Bisexual Women's Health

OFF AND ON I KEPT thinking. I have cancer. I'm a Black lesbian feminist poet, how am I going to do this now? Where are the models for what I'm supposed to be in this situation? But there were none. This is it, Audre. You're on your own. (Audre Lorde, 1980, pp. 28-29)

Most textbooks on women's health or obstetrics and gynecology ignore that 5%-10% of women are lesbian or bisexual (Dworkin & Gutierrez, 1989), or pay this fact lip service without considering its ramifications. Therefore, very little is known about the specific health problems of lesbians or bisexual women. Indeed, it is not known whether they do have any unique health needs. The following are some of the reasons for this lack of information:

- Lesbians and bisexual women are a largely invisible population. Unless a woman reveals her sexual identity to the health care provider, she remains hidden. Most caregivers assume that all their clients are heterosexual and many will claim that they have no lesbians or bisexuals in their practices.
- Heterosexism is the belief that heterosexuality is the only normal or natural option for women, and that heterosexuality is superior to lesbianism. Rather than respecting lesbians' and bisexual women's life choices and using affirmative research to improve the quality of care provided to them, investigators devalue or fail to consider lesbian and bisexual issues, or see nonheterosexual identities as diseases rather than as viable, acceptable identities. Rosser (1993) noted that lesbian health issues are "ignored, overlooked, or subsumed" (p. 183).

161

- Homophobia refers to negative attitudes about lesbians (or gay men), and biphobia refers to negative attitudes about bisexuals. Both can affect research in many ways. Some of the early research on lesbians has been biased by surveying lesbians in prisons or on psychiatric units and generalizing these findings to all lesbians, or by starting with the assumption that lesbians are deviates and conducting research to prove that point. Homophobia also contributes to the invisibility of lesbians because the negative attitudes are the primary reason that many lesbians do not reveal their sexual identity to caregivers. Still less attention has been paid to the needs of bisexual women—there is even very little "bad" research on bisexuals.

- The conservatism of research funding agencies is another factor. Until fairly recently, women in general were rarely the focus of health research and were often excluded from large-scale projects. Although investigators are beginning to include women in research samples, lesbian/bisexual women as a group are actively excluded or ignored because of political concerns (how would taxpayers react) or because of the misperception that it would be difficult to study such a small group (Rosser, 1993). Most research on women's health issues does, in fact, include lesbians and bisexual women, but these surveys or interviews seldom ask questions about sexual identity, obscuring potential differences between lesbians, bisexuals, and heterosexual women.

- Health care researchers assume that since lesbians and bisexuals are women, their issues and health needs are the same as those of heterosexual women. In the ideal, nonhomophobic world, this may be true. But the reality is that lesbians and bisexual women are treated differently from heterosexual women in society and within health care systems.

A major problem in studying lesbian and bisexual women's health is their diversity. The study of "lesbians" or "bisexuals" as monolithic groups is highly problematic (see, e.g., Anzaldua, 1987; Lim-Hing, 1994; Ramos, 1994; Roscoe, 1987; Silvera, 1991). There are few similarities among lesbians after accounting for choice of primary sexual/romantic partners. Bisexual women are even more diverse, as they may be in same-sex or other-sex primary relationships that, to the outside observer, sometimes resemble those of lesbians and other times, those of heterosexual women. Lesbians and bisexual women come from every racial/ethnic group, all socioeconomic classes, and all religions, geographic regions, national origins, types of family structures; and they suffer the same ailments and disabilities as the rest of the population. Because I must oversimplify and generalize the information in this chapter, you must take that factor into account when dealing with individual cases. The small amount of research into the health needs of lesbians or bisexual women has focused on White, well-educated, mostly middle-class, mostly lesbian women.

The label "lesbian" is itself a problem in studying lesbian health. Not all women who love other women identify with the label. Some women of color have objected to the term as a White, middle-class construct, or as an example of the Western world's insistence on categorizing and labeling (Mason-John & Khambatta, 1993). For others, lesbian is an uncomfortable word; "gay" comes easier. Older women who were socialized before the gay liberation movement may prefer to call themselves "gay women" or use a euphemism (Deevy, 1990). Some bisexual women in relationships with other women may be in "lesbian relationships," but do not consider themselves lesbians. Although less has been written about it, women who are behaviorally bisexual may be as diverse regarding the terms they choose to describe themselves as women who are behaviorally lesbians. With these limitations in mind, the following sections will review health concerns for lesbian and bisexual women.

Lesbian and Bisexual Women's Physical Health

Do adult lesbian and bisexual women differ from heterosexual women in the frequency or response to various reproductive transitions, such as pregnancy, infertility, or menopause? Do they have different risks for cancers or menstrual abnormalities? It appears that there are more similarities than differences, and that one of the major differences lies in access to quality health care. Lesbian and bisexual women, as a group, experience significantly greater barriers to health care, especially if they are poor, are from racial or ethnic minorities, or have a combination of these characteristics. There are two major categories of barriers (Eliason & Morgan, 1996c). First, there are financial concerns such as lack of domestic partner coverage in most areas of the United States, the fact that women still make less money than men make, resulting in a lesbian couple having measurably less disposable income than heterosexual or gay male couples, and the fact that women are more likely than men to work in jobs with no health benefits. Second, homophobia and heterosexism in health care providers and embedded in health care systems affect patient care. Health care providers vary widely in their attitudes about lesbians from acceptance to tolerance to disapproval, and even to disgust and hatred (Douglas, Kalman, & Kalman, 1985; Eliason, Donelan, & Randall, 1992; Eliason & Raheim, in press; Eliason & Randall, 1991; White, 1979). Chapter 5 reviewed the studies of health care provider attitudes; negative attitudes are a major reason lesbian and bisexual women often do not disclose their sexual identities to health care providers. Denenberg (1992) gave the following example:

Fran came out as a lesbian to her doctor when he was asking her about birth control. During the exam, when he was placing the speculum in her vagina, he was extremely rough and he used a size that was uncomfortable for her. When Fran complained, he said, "I'm just trying to change your mind." (p. 14)

A woman's choice not to disclose her sexual identity could lead to inappropriate treatment or teaching, or avoiding or delaying seeking health care for fear of poor treatment (Reagan, 1981). Such delays can have serious consequences, especially for medical problems that respond well to early treatment, such as cervical cancers and sexually transmitted infections.

Specific health issues of adult women include the frequency of regular gynecological care, sexually transmitted infections (STI) including HIV, cancers of reproductive organs and the breasts, sexual dysfunctions, and pregnancy-related issues. Each of these will be discussed separately.

Regular Gynecological Care

Buenting (1992) asked 27 lesbians and 52 heterosexual women to rate how central certain kinds of lifestyle factors were to their lives. Lesbians were significantly less likely to report that obtaining regular Pap smears were central. Indeed, Smith, Johnson, and Guenther (1985) found that lesbians were less likely to seek regular gynecological care—58% of their sample sought care only if they had a problem. Bradford and Ryan (1988) found that 50% of the lesbian and bisexual women in their sample had not had a Pap smear in the past year. Many women appear to believe that regular gynecological care is only necessary for obtaining birth control. And lesbians have often been harassed by health care providers about birth control issues. If the health care provider asks, "Are you sexually active?" a sexually active lesbian has to carefully consider the options. Either she comes out to the health care provider, lies and says "no," or says "yes" and gets a lecture about birth control. Most lesbians dislike being forced to disclose their sexual identity in this manner—they are comfortable disclosing it in their own way and in their own time (Reagan, 1981).

Trippet and Bain (1993) found that many lesbians sought self-care solutions or homeopathic remedies rather than mainstream health care. The main reasons for seeking traditional medical care were menstrual problems, sexually transmitted infections, and other reproductive problems (such as pelvic pain, uterine infections, painful sex, and lack of orgasms).

Eliason and Morgan (1996c) surveyed 101 lesbians aged 22–53 (mean age, 37), and found that 53% of their sample had a Pap smear in the past year, 29% in the past 1–2 years, 13% more than three years ago, and 5% had never had one. Breast self-exams were done frequently by 38% of the sample, but rarely by the rest. By age group, most of the women under the age of 40 had never had a mammogram (69%), whereas most of the women over 40 had undergone mammography (86%). Severe menstrual abnormalities were reported by 19% of the under-40s and 27% of the over-40s. Additionally, 13% had experienced an unwanted pregnancy at some time in their lives.

Most gynecologists who are knowledgeable about lesbian health issues recommend that lesbians have Pap smears at least every two years, and yearly if the person has any risk factor for cervical or breast cancer. Risks for cervical cancer include early age of first vaginal intercourse, multiple male sex partners, and history of sexually transmitted infections, especially human papilloma virus. Risk factors for breast cancer include smoking, heavy alcohol use, never having been pregnant or delaying pregnancy, and family history of breast cancer. Bisexual women should follow the guidelines for heterosexual women if they are sexually active with men.

Sexually Transmitted Infections Other Than HIV

Lesbians appear to have lower rates of gonorrhea, syphilis, pelvic inflammatory disease, and chlamydia than heterosexual or bisexual women, and about equivalent rates of vaginal yeast infections, human papilloma virus, and genital herpes as heterosexual and bisexual women (Johnson & Palermo, 1984; Johnson, Smith, & Guenther, 1987a; Robertson & Schachter, 1981). Degen and Waitkevicz (1982) studied the causes of vaginitis in 229 lesbians presenting with vaginal symptoms and found that the most common was a nonspecific vaginitis (39%), followed by vaginal candidiasis (24%), cervicitis (unspecified, 23%), and trichomonias (14%). These authors and others suggest that many sexually transmitted infections are acquired initially from heterosexual contact, but that most can be spread to female sexual partners.

Bisexual women in many studies are lumped with heterosexual women—in actuality, a careful history must be taken, as some bisexual women have very little heterosexual sexual contact. The client with an STI who is in a same-sex relationship may have different patient teaching needs from the heterosexual client, since the most common teaching for the heterosexual is "use a condom." A discussion of safer sex techniques for female sexual partners will follow the next section.

HIV/AIDS

In general, women with AIDS have been understudied, but empirical research on lesbians and AIDS is virtually nonexistent. Early in the epidemic, it was commonly thought that lesbians were at no risk for HIV infection because of several common stereotypes, primarily that women do not use IV drugs, and that lesbians and bisexual women are "less sexual" than gay men or heterosexuals (stemming from some people's belief that a penis must be present for sex to occur). When women began to test positive for HIV, they were reported to be mostly IV drug users or partners of male IV drug users. In 1984, Sabatini, Patel, and Hirschman reported what appears to be the first well-documented case of female-to-female transmission of HIV. Other reports followed (Marmor et al., 1986; Monzon & Capellan, 1987; Perry, Jacobsberg, & Fogel, 1989; Rich, Buck, Tuomala, & Kazanjian, 1993), mostly in the form of letters to medical journals. Chu, Buehler, Fleming, and Berkelman (1990) examined all cases of AIDS in women reported from 1980 to 1989 and found 79 women who reported exclusive sexual relations with women. Among this group, which was 42% Latina, 38% African American, and 19% European American, 95% were IV drug users. They also found 103 bisexual women, of whom 79% were IV drug users, 16% had male sex partners who were at high risk for or known to be HIV positive, and 4% had a history of blood transfusion. Chu et al. suggested, "Female-to-female transmission of HIV appears to be an extremely rare event" (p. 1381), and they called for increased efforts to prevent and reduce IV drug use in lesbians and bisexual women.

Two recent articles have challenged the notion that female-to-female transmission is "extremely rare." Stevens (1993a) noted several problems with the Center for Disease Control's (CDC) treatment of lesbians and HIV:

1. The CDC does not have a risk category for female-to-female transmission. A woman with no IV drug exposure, blood transfusion, or other blood sharing, and no male heterosexual contact is put under "no identified risk" or "other." If a lesbian has had any other risk factor (such as having sex once several years earlier with a man of unknown HIV status), she is reported under that risk category. Cole and Cooper (1990/1991) found that twice as many women as men are in this "other" category, suggesting different risk factors for women.

2. The most common manifestations of HIV in women are not listed in CDC's criteria for an AIDS diagnosis. These include vaginal candidias, pelvic inflammatory disease, human papilloma virus, genital herpes, and cervical dysplasia.

3. The CDC's definition of lesbian is too restrictive and does not reflect reality. The CDC defines a lesbian as a woman who has had sexual contact only with women since 1977. The reality is that most lesbians have had some sexual contact with men (75%–80%), and some lesbians continue to have occasional sexual encounters with men. None of these heterosexual experiences discount the possibility of HIV infection from a woman.

Stevens noted that these problems with the CDC's definitions and AIDS criteria result in a lack of safer sex education among lesbians, a false sense of security, and interference with early diagnosis and treatment. She comments:

The belief that "lesbians don't get AIDS," which is propagated by the CDC and the health professions . . . robs lesbians with HIV of a recognizable identity when they seek help. HIV-positive lesbians feel invisible in women's HIV support groups and other services that focus on heterosexual life experiences. They are alienated by HIV services for injection drug users that are not openly inclusive and sensitive to them. They report feeling as if they are the only women in a system of HIV services that are designed primarily for men. (p. 291)

Warren (1993) cited unpublished data from several medical centers that indicate that many HIV-positive women report a history of sexual activity with women (as many as 30%–40% of HIV-positive women). There is some indication that women who are risk takers in general—IV drug users, women who exchange sex for money or drugs—are also more likely to have sex with women (see also Bevier, Chiasson, Hefferman, & Castro, 1995). This subset of lesbian/bisexual women who use IV drugs need further study. Warren reported that 19%–32% of HIV-positive, IV-drug-using women consider themselves lesbian or bisexual. However, women with AIDS have not been studied to the same extent as men. Men are asked more detailed questions about the number and sex of their sexual partners and about specific sexual activities—women are rarely asked these questions.

Lesbians or bisexual women with AIDS have difficulty accessing services; they are often excluded from experimental drug trials, and many die of HIV-related illnesses before a diagnosis is even made. Women of color make up a disproportionate share of AIDS cases among women (52% of women with AIDS are African American and 21% are Latinas). Lesbians and bisexual women with AIDS react in diverse ways:

Disbelief

"I'm a gay woman, living with AIDS. Nobody out here believes I'm real," says Marlene, the mother of three, who has recently been released from jail. "I'm starting to doubt it myself." (Warren, 1993, p. 16)

Fear of Negative Attitudes and/or Discrimination

"I stopped going to that place [drug treatment center] because I didn't know what they would say in the group when I started talking about my [female] lover," Iris says. "For a while I just sat there saying nothing." (Warren, 1993, p. 16)

Lack of Information

As lesbians we can't get information about how to protect ourselves from sexually transmitted diseases. Whatever we learned about our bodies was oriented toward reproductive kinds of things. The orientation is completely toward heterosexuality. The only place women get any information about wellness is through family planning services. Lesbians have to filter it and always translate what nurses and doctors say to figure out what it means for lesbians. (Stevens, 1993a, p. 293)

Because lesbian and bisexual women's communities have been ignored in HIV/AIDS research, no prevention activities have targeted lesbian and bisexual women, leading many lesbian and bisexual women to believe that they are not vulnerable to HIV. The result is that some women continue to practice high-risk behaviors. Lesbians of color are at particular risk, as one Latina respondent noted:

We aren't getting knowledge to protect our health. There are no safe sex messages or education efforts geared toward lesbian communities. It's really an issue for lesbians of color. We don't have information. A lot of risky behavior goes on. A lot of us, sometimes we sleep with men. There is needle use, too. I'm afraid I'm going to test positive for HIV. And I don't have the money to pay for health care. (Stevens, 1993a, p. 150)

Lesbians are not immune to HIV. Specific behavioral risk factors need to be examined more closely, but female-to-female transmission of HIV is possible. The lack of safer sex education in lesbian and bisexual communities is appalling. Health care providers need to provide accurate and specific information to lesbian and bisexual clients and be attuned to the early symptoms of HIV illness in women. Additionally, lesbian and bisexual women in AIDS organizations are disproportionately involved as paid or volunteer caregivers of AIDS patients. These roles are difficult and stressful.

Safer sex for women in same-sex relationships includes use of a barrier (e.g., a latex condom cut open, a dental dam, or a piece of plastic wrap) to avoid oral contact with vaginal fluids, menstrual blood, or other body fluids. If a woman has cuts or abrasions on her hands, she should use a glove or finger cot to avoid contact with body fluids. Women should not share sex toys (Rankow, 1995).

Cancers

Rates of some kinds of cancer, such as breast cancer, which is associated with lack of childbearing and breast feeding, may be higher in childless lesbians (Winnow, 1989/1990), whereas other kinds such as cervical cancer, which is associated with heterosexual vaginal intercourse, may be lower in lesbians (Johnson & Palermo, 1984; however, 75%–80% of lesbians have had some degree of heterosexual sexual experience, which may increase their risk). There has not been sufficient research to support these hypotheses at this time. Since many types of cancer are also associated with stress, lesbians may be at higher risk because the homophobia in society increases stress in the workplace, home, and everyday life. As we have already seen, many lesbians delay seeking health care, contributing to poorer outcomes when they do develop a cancer.

Eliason and Morgan (1996c) surveyed 101 lesbians and found that 3% of the women over 40 had breast cancer compared with none of the under-40 group. Cystic breast disease was fairly common in both groups: 17% of the under-40 group and 24% of the over-40s. Cervical or uterine cancer was reported by none of the under-40s, but 11% of the over-40s. One risk factor for cancer is smoking: 9% of the under-40 and 16% of the over-40 group smoked. Another risk factor for some cancers is lack of pregnancy or childbearing: Over 80% of these women had not borne children.

Heavy alcohol use is another risk factor for many types of cancer and will be discussed later in this chapter. It appears that sexual identity per se is not the major consideration in assessing a woman's risk for cancer (or HIV or other STIs)—health care providers need to assess individual risk factors.

When a woman has cancer of any kind, partner support is crucial to her recovery, although health care providers often do not recognize or validate these relationships:

After Sonja's surgery for breast cancer, her lover Michelle was not allowed into the recovery room. As she sat in the waiting room for three hours, Michelle noted the nurses escorting other people in to see family members. She was afraid to complain, lest they treat Sonja badly. (Denenberg, 1992, p. 15)

So I went in with her [to the exam room] and I was completely discounted . . . she couldn't understand why I was there. She asked me about three times why I was there. It was harder for me to help her than probably it would have been if I had been a man sitting there with her and had a legitimate relationship to this person. (Robertson, 1992, p. 70)

Because lesbian and bisexual women lack support when they have cancer, several organizations have emerged in larger cities to provide support and education for women with cancer and their partners (see Denenberg, 1992). Until empirical studies are conducted on the rates of cancer in lesbian and bisexual women, all women should follow the same general guidelines for cancer detection and prevention. Eliminating factors that can increase the risk for cancer should be encouraged in all women; these include smoking, heavy alcohol use, obesity, and high cholesterol levels.

Sexual Dysfunctions

Some early literature on lesbians suggested that sexual dysfunctions were rare. For example, Kinsey's data from the 1950s suggested that lesbians were much more likely to be orgasmic than heterosexual women (Kinsey, Pomeroy, Martin, & Gebhard, 1953). More recent data, however, suggest that some lesbians have sexual problems, though the rates may be lower than in married heterosexual women (Johnson & Palermo, 1984). As a group, lesbian and bisexual women—like all women—have a high frequency of experiences of childhood sexual abuse and sexual coercion (Brannock & Chapman, 1990; Peters & Cantrell, 1991). Lesbian and bisexual women are also socialized into a culture that objectifies women's bodies and establishes a largely unattainable ideal of female beauty. These cultural ideals make many women hate or feel uncomfortable with their own bodies and sexuality. Women are also socialized to be passive in sexual relationships and to believe that men should initiate sex. Thus, women in relationships together may have more difficulty knowing how to initiate sex and may wait for the other to do the initiating (Loulan, 1984). Early socialization experiences, as well as incest, rape, or other traumas can affect adult sexual relationships in a variety of ways. In addition, internalized homophobia can affect lesbian sexual relationships if one or both partners feel any sense of guilt or shame about the relationship (Clunis & Green, 1993).

Pregnancy-Related Issues

> *A 41-year-old single, nulliparous woman came to the Fertility Center requesting an in vitro fertilization procedure with, possibly, an egg donation also. The patient presented herself without a partner, and although sexual orientation was never directly addressed, the physician observed indications that she was a lesbian. . . . In this particular situation, the physician refused to conduct the procedure itself because "the patient is single and questionably lesbian." (Curtin, 1994, p. 14)*

Estimating the number of lesbian mothers is difficult because the population is invisible. Some have suggested that about one-third of older lesbians have children from previous heterosexual relationships, whereas among younger lesbians, children come from donor insemination, adoption, and brief heterosexual encounters for the sole purpose of pregnancy as well as from previous heterosexual relationships (Pollach & Vaughn, 1987). Chapter 4 discussed some of the psychological and societal issues that lesbian parents face.

Johnson, Smith, and Guenther (1987b) asked 1,921 lesbians and 424 bisexual women about their parenting desires. More than half (an equal number of lesbians and bisexuals) had considered having a child since coming out (15% had a child from a previous heterosexual relationship). The preferred methods of obtaining a child were somewhat different for lesbian and bisexual women. Bisexual women said that they would seek intercourse with a cooperative man (65%), adopt (53%), or choose donor insemination (38%). Lesbians were nearly evenly split between adoption (62%) and donor insemination (61%), although 37% said they would choose intercourse with a cooperative man. Only 2% of the sample had achieved success in becoming a parent, and most of those did so via intercourse with an unsuspecting man (50%), intercourse with a cooperative man (39%), donor insemination (33%), and adoption (8%). This study indicated a large discrepancy between the number of women who desired parenting versus those who succeeded in becoming parents.

Lesbian and bisexual women need to be counseled that donor insemination and pregnancy by brief heterosexual encounters carry risk for HIV and other STIs. Women considering donor insemination should carefully screen sperm banks and only consider those that do careful history, physical assessment, and HIV testing of donors.

Lesbian and bisexual women considering parenting options should also be counseled about the potential effects of alcohol and drug use on fetal development. The relatively high rates of alcohol and drug consumption among lesbians pose a significant fetal risk, and as mentioned earlier, a number of lesbians have heterosexual experiences and may have unwanted pregnancies as well as planned pregnancies.

Health care providers may need to counsel prospective female same-sex couples seeking pregnancy or adoption to file appropriate legal papers to protect their families, including wills, durable power of attorney for health care, and papers conferring medical authority over the children to the nonbiological parent (Rankow, 1995).

When a woman in a primary relationship with another woman becomes pregnant, the couple may face developmental transitions that aid in adapting to the new motherhood role. Wismont and Reame (1989) explore some of the ways that health care providers can help lesbian couples adapt to pregnancy.

LESBIAN AND BISEXUAL WOMEN'S MENTAL HEALTH

Relatively more research has been done on mental health problems of lesbian and bisexual women than on physical health, partly because of societal stereotypes that lesbianism and bisexuality are mental illnesses. As discussed in Chapter 2, however, there is no evidence that sexual identity causes mental health symptoms. What does cause problems for lesbians and bisexual women is the daily stress of dealing with social stigma and internalized homophobia. Gillow and Davis (1987) surveyed 142 lesbians and found that most of the stress they experienced was caused by or exacerbated by being lesbians. The most common stressor they reported was job-related (27% of the sample). For example, one woman noted, "I am an elementary school teacher and I worry that when I have a teaching job my sexuality will become known and my job will be in danger" (p. 29). Other stressors included relationships (25%), such as the pressures of being in a stigmaticized relationship; family of origin problems (11%), such as rejection from parents or pressure to marry; and financial worries (10%). Lesbians with good social support networks had more adaptive coping strategies than those without good support. The most commonly used strategies to cope with stress included looking for the humor in the situation (94%), crying (92%), temporarily withdrawing from the situation (89%), and talking to someone (48–63%). However, nonadaptive coping strategies were also used: 59% drank alcohol as a response to stress and 32% used recreational drugs.

The largest study to date on lesbians and mental health was reported by Bradford, Ryan, and Rothblum (1994). They distributed surveys across the country and obtained a return rate of 42%, resulting in 1,925 completed surveys from lesbians from all 50 states. Compared with the 1980 U.S. Census data, the lesbian sample was more educated, younger, and more likely to be employed in a professional or managerial position than the general female population. The racial composition was similar, except that the lesbian sample contained fewer African Americans than the census data indicated. The section on mental health showed that the major concerns of lesbians in this sample were money (57%), job or school worries (31%), relationship problems (27%), and family problems (21%). Only 12% worried about people knowing that they were lesbians, but many were not out to all family or coworkers (especially Latina and African American lesbians). More African American lesbians worried about money (79%) than European American lesbians (56%) or Latina lesbians (57%). Although lifetime rates of depression were relatively high (37%), only 11% were currently in treatment for depression. Nearly 20% reported problems with anxiety in the past, and 7% were currently in treatment for anxiety. Twenty-one percent had suicidal thoughts sometimes or often, and 18% had attempted suicide at least once. African American and Latina lesbians were more likely to have attempted suicide than European American lesbians (27% African American, 28% Latina, 16% European American). Older women reported lower rates of depression, anxiety, and suicidal thoughts than younger women. Some of the depression, suicide, and anxiety at younger ages stemmed from experiences of abuse, as 37% of the sample had experienced at least one episode of physical abuse (24% while growing up and 16% as adults) and 41% had experienced sexual abuse (21% while growing up and 15% as adults). Rates of physical and sexual abuse (including incest) were higher in African American and Latina lesbians than European American lesbians.

Many lesbians in the sample had experienced discrimination due to their sexual identities; 52% had been verbally harassed, 8% had lost jobs, 6% had been physically attacked, and 1% had been discharged from the military. Only one lesbian in the sample had AIDS (data were collected in the early 1980s), but 60% reported that AIDS had greatly affected their lives, and 40% were worried about gay male friends.

Over 70% had received some form of professional counseling in the past or currently, and 36% had sought help from nonprofessionals such as friends, peer counselors, or support groups. European American lesbians were more likely to have received professional counseling (74%) than Latina or African American lesbians (61% for each group). The most frequently cited reason for counseling was depression (50%), followed by problems with lovers (44%), problems with family (34%), anxiety and fears (31%), loneliness (21%), and desire for personal growth (30%). A few cited being gay, racism, and alcohol and drug problems as reasons for therapy. This high rate of therapy usage among lesbian and bisexual women has been confirmed by several other studies (e.g., Eliason & Morgan, 1996b; Morgan, 1992; Morgan & Eliason, 1992). European American lesbian and bisexual women often value therapy as a means for personal growth, and lesbian communities often encourage therapy. Less is known about the use of therapy by lesbian and bisexual women of color—it is likely that they are more suspicious of mental health services because of the racism, sexism, and heterosexism that they face.

Bradford, Ryan, and Rothblum's report showed the potential mental health consequences of societal stigma, and the need for health care providers and mental health counselors to be aware of lesbian and bisexual issues and concerns. In the following sections, I will examine some of the most common mental health risks of lesbian and bisexual women: substance abuse, depression and suicide, eating disorders, and hate crimes.

Substance Abuse and Misuse

It is common to read that lesbians and bisexual women are at high risk for alcohol and drug abuse. Saghir and Robins (1973) reported that 35% of the lesbians in their sample had current or past alcohol problems, compared with only 5% of heterosexual women. Fifield (1975) found a rate of 25%. For nearly 20 years, these figures were repeated without question, and it was assumed that the social stigma of being lesbian or bisexual, combined with the central role of gay bars in lesbian, gay, and bisexual communities, led to the high rate. However, these early studies had very small and generally nonrepresentative samples. Recent data are challenging these old figures.

Bloomfield (1993) conducted a study with sound methodological characteristics. She began with a random sample of 4,000 San Francisco households and sent out questionnaires to all that were personal residences. She obtained a return rate of 23%, with 445 women responding. Eighty-five percent were primarily or exclusively heterosexual and 15% ($n = 58$) were lesbian or bisexual. There were no differences by sexual identity group on any of the self-report measures of drinking patterns, such as the number of abstainers, light drinkers, and heavy drinkers, except for one category. More lesbian and bisexual women were in the category labeled "recovering alcoholic." In the lesbian and bisexual group, 13% considered themselves to be recovering alcoholics compared with only 3% of the heterosexual women. There were no differences in the number who drank more than 60 drinks in the past 30 days, the mean number of drinks per month or day, or the mean number of drinking days. Multiple regression analyses found only one significant predictor of heavy alcohol use: bar going, regardless of sexual identity. Bloomfield suggested that the higher number of recovering alcoholics in the lesbian and bisexual sample may be due to the increased awareness of alcohol and drug problems that occurred in many lesbian/bisexual communities in the 1980s, as well as the increase in alternatives to bars for women's socializing. Thus, the finding of higher numbers of heavy drinking or alcoholic lesbians and bisexual women in the earlier studies reflected nonrepresentative samples, the historical importance of gay bars in the 1950s and 1960s, and changes in awareness and attitudes about drinking since that time. Thus, heavy drinking may be a more significant problem for the older generation of lesbian and bisexual women. Eliason and Morgan (1996c) found that 5% of lesbians under 40 drank daily whereas 14% of lesbians over 40 drank daily.

Many studies also report higher drug use in lesbian and bisexual women than in the general population of women. McKirnan and Peterson (1989a) surveyed 3,400 lesbian, gay, and bisexual residents of Chicago, recruited from a gay newspaper and several gay organizations and community events. There were 748 lesbian and bisexual women with a mean age of 32 (88% White). Most of the women were in stable relationships (65%), and 11% reported that they were out to no one or only one person. Table 7.1 shows drug use patterns for the lesbian/bisexual group compared with the general population of women. Although lesbian/bisexual women had much higher lifetime prevalence rates of marijuana and cocaine, their frequent use patterns were not very different from the general population.

TABLE 7.1.   Lifetime and Frequent Use of Marijuana and Cocaine in 748 Lesbian and Bisexual Women Compared with General Population Rates for Women, by Age Group

	General Population (%)	Lesbian/Bisexual (%)
Lifetime Use of Marijuana		
18-25	60	85
26-34	47	88
35+	7	67
Frequent Use of Marijuana		
18-25	9	11
26-34	7	14
35+	.2	6
Lifetime Use of Cocaine		
18-25	22	57
26-34	18	51
35+	2	23
Frequent Use of Cocaine		
18-25	.3	3.3
26-34	.2	1.8
35+	0	.9

Note. Adapted from McKirnan and Peterson (1989a).

Skinner (1994) surveyed 190 lesbians with a mean age of 36.4, who were 92% White. Skinner asked about a wide variety of licit and illicit drugs as well as alcohol. Table 7.2 shows the prevalence of drug use in the month prior to the survey, divided by age group. Lesbians in this sample had an appallingly high rate of cigarette and alcohol use, but only small minorities of lesbians used other types of drugs. Demographic variables did not predict drug use very well—marijuana use was associated with younger age, and cigarette use was associated with lower education; however, none of the demographic variables predicted alcohol use.

Alcohol or drug problems of lesbians and bisexual women may be related to the individual's childhood experiences such as having an alcoholic parent or having more unhappy and conflictual relationships with parents, and having less social support as an adult (Schilit, Clark, & Shallenberger, 1988). Close friends who are heavy drinkers provide role models for drinking and weaken the social support needed to stop drinking (Weinberg, 1994).

Joanne Hall (1994) interviewed 35 lesbians who were in long-term recovery from alcohol (24 European Americans, 6 African Americans, 3

TABLE 7.2.   Licit and Illicit Drug Use in 190 Lesbians in the Month
Prior to the Survey

| | Age Group | | |
Drug	18-25	26-34	35+
Marijuana	24%	21%	14%
Cocaine	0	5	2
Crack	0	0	0
Inhalants	6	3	3
Hallucinogens	0	5	0
Heroin	0	0	0
Stimulants	0	3	0
Sedatives	0	2	0
Tranquilizers	2	2	2
Analgesics	0	0	0
Psychotherapeutics	0	3	2
Alcohol	77	67	63
Cigarettes	53	44	38

Note. Adapted from Skinner (1994).

Latinas, 1 Asian Pacific-Islander, 1 Native American). The mean age of
the women was 37, and they had a mean income of $27,000, which was
below the San Francisco mean income of $30,000, even though 60% had
college degrees. The drinking and drug histories of these women revealed that 91% abused alcohol and drugs, 34% had compulsive food
habits, and 63% had received formal treatment for their substance abuse.
Nearly all of them had received individual counseling for their substance
abuse and 77% had participated in group therapy. Sixty-three percent
had been abused as children; 46% had been sexually abused.

Hall identified three barriers to effective treatment for lesbians
with substance abuse problems: (1) client's distrust, (2) provider-
client incongruence, and (3) health care provider style. Each of these
barriers will be discussed, along with some examples of lesbians' actual experiences.

Client's Distrust of Providers.   In most cases, lesbians worried or perceived that their providers did not understand sexuality issues, or they
felt discriminated against on the basis of gender, race, ethnicity, sexuality, or social class. Some noted that health care providers' heterosexist assumptions got in the way, and others noted that health care

providers reacted negatively to their disclosure as lesbians. Some were told not to disclose in their group therapy sessions, and others felt unsafe to disclose:

> *I had a lot of problems. But I couldn't let the counselors into my world. It was clear from the way they talked that they were homophobic. And they let the other patients say that stuff, too. It made me really vulnerable. I thought, oh, they are leaving it to me to educate them. No way. I mean it wasn't even safe to be there. (Hall, 1994, p. 240)*

Health Care Provider–Client Conceptual Congruence.   This factor was the degree to which client and provider matched on their definitions of the problem and their approach to treatment. Most of the incongruence came from providers who lacked knowledge about race, gender, or sexuality.

Health Care Provider Persuasive Styles.   Hall found four different styles of health care provider interactions with clients.

1. *Paternalistic:*

    I had attempted suicide and I told the psychiatrist, "I'm gay, I'm 18. I'm scared." On the third appointment, he said, "Next time you come in to see me, I want you to wear a dress." I was taken aback. He thought that if I changed my clothes and put on a little makeup I would feel like a "girl" again. I never returned, and it was many years before I sought help again. (Hall, 1994, pp. 241–242)

2. *Maternalistic.* This approach was considered positive by many clients who needed some nurturance and support.

3. *Confrontational.* This style caused the most difficulty for lesbian clients.

    In inpatient treatment they escorted me to AA [Alcoholics Anonymous]. I didn't want to go. . . . What if they have a problem with lesbians at the meeting? To be force-fed AA felt like I was being pushed into the closet, to make me straight and Christian. (Hall, 1994, p. 242)

4. *Influential.* This approach involved a safe, accepting environment where client and provider negotiated treatment, and where

challenging unhealthy beliefs or behaviors was balanced with
emotional support:

> It's hard enough to be a lesbian, making it in society. When
> you also have a booze or drug problem, you are vulnerable
> to that negative image of lesbians being drunks. All that
> keeps you from getting help. One nurse in the treatment
> center showed me respect by giving me options. She bent
> the rules. She told me not to throw any parts of myself
> away. I learned from her that I could recover from my
> drinking problem and still be a lesbian, and that being a les-
> bian was a good thing. (Hall, 1994, p. 243)

Hall concluded from her data that AA may not always be the best
choice for women, especially lesbians and women of color, because the
AA themes of powerlessness, surrender, and belief in a higher power
may be "culturally and politically dissonant" (1994, p. 243). Glaus
(1989) agreed that the low self-esteem, shame, and guilt in many female alcoholics may render AA inappropriate.

Schilit, Lie, and Montagne (1990) explored the connections between
substance abuse and domestic violence in 104 lesbians (93% European
American, 2% Latina, 1% African American, 1% Native American). In this
sample, 8% of the women drank every day, and 27% drank 2–6 times per
week. Slightly fewer used drugs regularly: Just under 8% used some drug
daily and 35% used some drug once a week or less. Marijuana was the
most often used drug (43% had used it at some time), followed by
hashish (11%) and antianxiety drugs (10%). Thirty-nine women reported currently being in a abusive relationship. Of that group, 64% of
the respondents reported using drugs or alcohol prior to battering
episodes. The authors did not ask whether the respondent was being battered or doing the battering, and a cross-sectional study cannot tell us
whether substance abuse causes domestic violence. This study, however, like many others, suggests a link between substance abuse and domestic violence. Less than half of the women in abusive relationships
had sought help. Of those who did seek help, only one went to a battered
women shelter and 18 sought counseling. Chapter 4 discussed some of
the barriers to treatment for battered lesbians.

Thus, a significant number of lesbian and bisexual women have alcohol or drug dependencies, although the actual percentage is ap-
proaching that of the general population of women. When lesbian and

bisexual women require help for their substance abuse, they often encounter hostile or nonsupportive systems and health care providers.

Depression and Suicide

Although many early studies reported no significant differences between heterosexuals and lesbian, gay, and bisexual people on personality or psychological adjustment measures, they did report slight elevations on depression scales and a higher lifetime prevalence of depressive symptoms. Rothblum (1990) noted that studies of depression in general have documented higher rates of depression in women than men, often rates that are twice as high. As women, lesbians have some of the same risk and protective factors as heterosexual women such as social support, intimate relationships, mothering, and employment. In addition, they have risk factors such as alienation from heterosexual society, the stresses of coming out, and degree of integration into lesbian communities. Rothblum noted that European American lesbians are 2½ times more likely than European American heterosexual women to attempt suicide. Table 7.3 lists the lifetime and/or current rates of

TABLE 7.3.   Rates of Depression among Lesbian and Bisexual Women

Authors	Sample	Findings*
Saghir, Robins, Walbran, & Gentry (1970b)	57 lesbians	44% lifetime
	43 hetero. women	35% lifetime
Johnson, Guenther, Laube, & Keettell (1981)	117 lesbians	30% lifetime
Saunders, Tupac, & MacCullouch (1988)	996 lesbians	49% lifetime
Trippet & Bain (1990)	42 lesbians, 1 bisexual	65% lifetime
Bradford, Ryan & Rothblum (1994)	1,925 lesbians	37% lifetime
		11% current
Cochran & Mays (1994)	603 African American lesbians and bisexuals	38% current
Trippet (1994)	503 lesbians	66% lifetime
Eliason & Morgan (1996c)	101 lesbians	59% lifetime

* Lifetime = ever experienced significant depressive symptoms. Current = currently experiencing significant depressive symptoms.

depression in some of the studies that have examined depression in lesbian and/or bisexual women.

Cochran and Mays (1994) suggested that African American lesbians and bisexual women are at particularly high risk for depression because of the intersections of racism, sexism, and heterosexism. They conducted a national survey of homosexually active African American women and men. There were 603 female respondents (84% lesbian, 11% bisexual, and 5% who did not identify as either, but were sexually active with women), with a mean age of 33. The women, as a group, reported a high number of depressive symptoms on the Center for Epidemiologic Studies Depression Scale (CES-D). In fact, they scored higher than most of the African American gay and bisexual men, even those with AIDS. Their mean score of 14.7 was just under the cutoff score of 15 that indicates potentially clinically significant depression, and 38% scored higher than 15. The authors concluded that the combined effects of race, sex, and sexual identity result in African American lesbian and bisexual women having more problems with depressive symptoms than heterosexual African American women and men, or African American gay and bisexual men. Despite the higher prevalence rates of depression, African American lesbian and bisexual women may not seek treatment because of the cost, the stigma associated with psychological or psychiatric treatment, and fear of prejudicial treatment by counselors.

Eating Disorders

Siever (1994) found that, in general, lesbians were more satisfied with their bodies and less vulnerable to eating disorders than were heterosexual women, presumably because heterosexual women are motivated to attract and please heterosexual men who place value on women's physical appearance, and because advertising and other forms of media stress slenderness as being "feminine." Nevertheless, individual lesbians have problems with body image: some stem from earlier life experiences of trying to fit into a heterosexual woman's mold; others stem from dysfunctional responses to internalized homophobia or experiences of oppression (Thompson, 1994). Thompson interviewed women who were African American, Latina, working class, and/or lesbians—groups thought to be less susceptible to eating disorders than White middle-class heterosexual young women. One of her informants,

Jackie, a 28-year-old White lesbian, developed bulimia as a teenager at the same time she felt confusion about her sexuality. She noted: "I was not being a social, effective heterosexual kid and could not identify in that way, could not imagine being somebody's girlfriend. . . . Maybe I could be a more successful heterosexual if I were skinnier" (Thompson, 1994, p. 81).

Once this informant began to acknowledge her lesbian identity, the binge-purge cycle began to subside. Lesbian and bisexual women may be recovering from eating disorders or still actively engaging in unhealthy eating patterns. Eliason and Morgan (1996c) found that 25% of the lesbians in their sample reported some type of eating disorder in their lives (including anorexia, bulimia, and compulsive overeating). Eating disorders are a complex response to stressful situations, past or present, in women's lives. A woman who feels powerless over other aspects of her life (e.g., racism, sexism, heterosexism) may focus on one of the few areas over which she has total control—what and how she eats (McClure & Vespry, 1994).

Hate Crimes

It was May 13, 1988, the second day of a three-day backpacking trip on the Appalachian Trail in south-central Pennsylvania. . . . We had no premonition, no warning that the world as we knew it was about to be irreparably shattered. . . . Even our two brief exchanges with the stranger on the trail, though disturbing, had seemed of little consequence. . . . We thought he was a strange character, a "creep," but we had no clues that he was planning to murder us. No clue that, after we saw him continue south on the trail, as we headed east on a side trail, he would circle back around to ensure that our paths intersected once again, this time with him hidden. From that position, on a glorious sunny Friday afternoon, he lay with his rifle. After he watched us make love and have fun, he exploded our world with his hate and his bullets [Claudia was seriously injured but walked four miles in the dark for help; her partner, Rebecca, died of her injuries]. (Claudia Brenner, 1992, pp. 12-13)

Lesbian and bisexual women, like gay and bisexual men, are often targeted for violence, solely on the basis of their sexual identities. Von Schulthess (1992) surveyed 400 lesbian and bisexual women from San

Francisco (82% White, 6% African American, 5% Latina, 2% Asian American, and 2% Native American). Most were between the ages of 20 and 35 (78%). Over their lifetimes, 40% had been threatened with physical violence; 33% had someone chase or follow them; 27% had objects thrown at them; 12% had been punched, hit, kicked, or beaten; 6% had been sexually assaulted or raped; and 3% had been assaulted with a weapon—all because of their perceived sexual identities. Only 15% of those victimized had reported it to the police. Lesbians of color experienced higher rates of physical violence, threats, vandalism, and rape than White lesbians. Many of the women in the sample said that their victimization was a combination of sexism and heterosexism that was often difficult to sort out. Many reported daily harassment because they were women. The author noted:

> *Men expect women to act in certain ways in response to their "come-on." Carol Brooks Gardner (1980, p. 346), who had done research on street remarks, suggests that "retaliation is not considered feminine behavior." A woman who answers back or does something that is construed as retaliation is seen by her assailant as nonfeminine and therefore as engaging in behavior that is inappropriate for her gender. If the assailant is unhappy with the victim's response, one way of escalating the attack is to shift the harassment from antiwoman to antilesbian commentary. (von Schulthess, 1992, pp. 70-71)*

In general, men and women experience slightly different varieties of hate crimes. Berrill (1992) reported that men experience more harassment, threats, and physical violence from nonfamily members and in public gay-identified areas. Women experience more verbal harassment from family members, are discriminated against more often than gay men, and are victimized in nongay identified public areas and in the home. Berrill (1992) also confirmed that lesbian, gay, and bisexual people of color are victimized more often than Whites.

INTERVIEWING LESBIAN AND BISEXUAL
FEMALE CLIENTS OR PATIENTS

Lynch (1993) suggested the following helpful interview techniques. They can be used with all clients, but are inclusive of lesbian and bisexual women as well as heterosexual women who live with a sexual partner to whom they are not married:

1. Instead of the usual marital status question, ask questions such as:

     With whom do you live?

     Who is important to you?

     Do you live with your sexual partner?

2. "Sexual partner" is a gender-neutral term as opposed to "boy-friend" or "husband."

3. Regarding sexual activity, health care providers could ask:

     Do you practice safe sex with all your partners?

     What precautions do you use?

4. Use specific terms like oral sex, vaginal sex, and anal sex instead of the vague "sex" or "intercourse."

Lucas (1992) found that 64% of the lesbians in her study wanted health care providers to ask directly about sexual identity, but only 28% wanted it on their medical records. In Chapter 9, I will describe some additional ways to ask about sexual identity.

In many health care settings that women use a major question is, "Are you sexually active?" Robertson (1992) provided some examples of lesbians' experiences with that question:

I might have said yes [to being sexually active] and they said do you need birth control. I said no. Maybe they were a little con-fused. I could have also said no, thinking, well it's not real sex, you know, to them.

I think it just confused them. I remember they just didn't be-lieve me when I said I was sexually active but I wasn't using birth control.

In answering the questions, are you sexually active and do you use birth control, I just write down I'm a lesbian and that they are very heterosexist questions and that they need to change their questionnaire. (Robertson, 1992, p. 69)

Lesbian and bisexual women tend to avoid traditional health care systems whenever possible because of past bad experiences, financial difficulties, and the expectation that they will receive poor care. Trippet and Bain (1993) suggested that health care systems need to make some systematic changes to accommodate the needs of lesbian and bisexual women:

- *Practice Changes.* Provide more holistic care, include natural remedies, and focus on education and prevention.
- *Practical Changes.* Decrease cost, increase availability, include insurance coverage for alternative treatments, develop increased (and better) communication skills.

Lucas (1992) and many others have found that lesbian and bisexual women tend to prefer women as their health care providers, whether physicians, physician assistants, nurse practitioners, or midwives. Health care settings need to allow patients or clients the right to choose their primary health care provider.

CONCLUSION

Although there is greater acknowledgment of the need to understand and include lesbian and bisexual women in health care, the literature continues to include unscientific and biased information. As a profession, we need to demand higher standards and refuse to print articles that are based on personal opinion or that are contrary to the bulk of scientific research. We allow the freedom of speech in our society, but our professional journals must have scientific standards. One such example of unscientific reports comes from the 1992 issue of the *Journal of Christian Nursing.* An article by Elizabeth Moberly, founder of one of the many "reparative" therapies to cure homosexuality, cites "evidence" of the origin of homosexuality in dysfunctional families. Moberly urges gay men to become more masculine and lesbians to become more feminine as a means of overcoming homosexuality. The other article is a painful account of an "ex-lesbian" who was "cured" by Exodus International, another reparative therapy organization. The author notes that she still feels attractions for women, and writes:

I am now able to catch myself before I get carried away in my thoughts. I have better discernment as to when my thoughts are

*progressing from pondering something to sin. I still have diffi-
culties in this area. Evil can become deeply entrenched in the
mind. However, I am experiencing progressive freedom as I sin-
cerely ask God to change me to hate this sin and teach me how
to combat it in his power. (Young, 1992, p. 13)*

It is so unfortunate that this young woman has been taught to hate a
powerful part of her self and to feel guilt over her attractions (which
could not be altered by therapy or prayer). Health care professions need
to find ways to alleviate pain and suffering, not to compound them.

EXERCISE: IS YOUR OWN
ORGANIZATION INCLUSIVE?

Consider your own work setting. How could you make it more inclusive
of lesbian, gay, and bisexual clients or patients? What would you need to
change (consider written forms, interview techniques, policies, and procedures)? What kind of resistance might you meet if you suggested a
change?

Chapter Eight

Gay and Bisexual Men's Health

I LEARNED I WAS HIV-positive in 1987. I've probably been seropositive for longer than that. I've outlasted my lovers, my friends, some of my exes, my tricks, my relatives, even some of the queens I couldn't stand. I've outlasted our doctor. I've even outlasted the guilt of still being alive and healthy. It's funny. There is no satisfaction in that word: outlasted. There is no satisfaction in living longer than friends and loved ones. No catharsis crying at yet another memorial service. I don't go to them anymore. The miracle of survival. Survival is a spot between the rock of guilt and the hard place of memory. (Robert Vasquez-Pacheco, 1993, p. 81)

Since the early 1980s, the major health concern for gay and bisexual men has been HIV and AIDS. A literature search on homosexuality and health reveals virtually thousands of entries about AIDS. An in-depth presentation of AIDS care and prevention is beyond the scope of this book, but I will explore a few key themes in this chapter, including the phobic attitudes of health care providers toward homosexuality and AIDS, and how these attitudes impact patient care and prevention activities; the need for all health care providers to learn how to interview about sexuality and sexual behavior; and the role of health care providers in providing safer-sex education.

Other potential health risks for gay and bisexual men have been somewhat ignored in recent years because of the understandably inordinate focus on AIDS. These include mental health problems related to hate crimes, or violence directed at men who are perceived to be gay or bisexual. In addition, internalized homophobia can manifest as low self-esteem, depression and suicide, substance abuse, and domestic violence.

Although such problems can also stem from other factors—dysfunctional childhood experiences, depressing life events, and psychiatric illnesses—they often are compounded by societal stigma and homophobia. Physical health concerns include sexually transmitted infections other than HIV and related medical conditions that result from an active sexual life.

GAY AND BISEXUAL MEN'S MENTAL HEALTH

As I have noted repeatedly, belonging to an oppressed minority group can put incredible stress on the individual. Management of this stress depends on a multitude of factors including, but not limited to, individual coping strategies and personality style, the amount and quality of social support, acceptance of sexual identity, the presence of a stable relationship, and general health. Fear and anxiety about HIV/AIDS, or living with HIV/AIDS, are major sources of stress for gay and bisexual men today. I will explore just a few of the mental health problems that can arise from being a gay or bisexual man in contemporary U.S. society.

Hate Crimes

Paul Cotton (1992) reported the following case study in the *Journal of the American Medical Association:*

> *Paul Carson, MD, says he "couldn't conceive of anybody doing" what his patient claims to have done. The patient, a married heterosexual truck driver, insists that his only risk for acquiring his human immunodeficiency virus (HIV) infection was cuts on his hands during the many bloody beatings he and friends systematically inflicted on randomly selected gay men over several years, "too many times to count." "It was a sort of diversion, entertainment with friends, and they [gay men] were easy targets." (p. 2999)*

Reports of "gay-bashing" incidents have increased in the 1990s, partly due to public resentment and fears about AIDS, and partly due to the greater visibility of lesbian, gay, and bisexual people in society. Cotton reported that hate crimes against lesbian, gay, and bisexual people are more than random violence. The attackers are often armed with crowbars, chains, clubs, and baseball bats, and they outnumber their victims or take them by surprise. Like perpetrators of racial violence, gay-bashers consider themselves to be enforcing societal norms and defending "their own kind." Unlike perpetrators of racial violence, who often beat the person of color who inadvertently enters the wrong neighborhood or the wrong bar, gay-bashers often go into gay neighborhoods seeking out their victims. Gay-bashers are most often adolescents, and/or middle-class adults who can afford lawyers. They generally have no prior police records and judges are notoriously lenient with them. Gay-bashers are often seen as "justified" in their attacks by claiming that the victim "hit on" them. This so-called homosexual panic defense has been used across the country to get lighter sentences for gay-bashers, some of whom have murdered their victims in brutal fashion.

One early example of the leniency of judges and juries to gay-bashers is the case of Dan White. In 1978, White, a former San Francisco supervisor, climbed in a back window of the City Hall with a loaded revolver and several extra clips of ammunition. He shot and killed Harvey Milk, the first openly gay elected official in the country, and mayor George Moscone. White was convicted of manslaughter rather than first degree murder and sentenced to seven years in prison: He served only five years. Many political commentators believe that his sentence was so light because one of his victims was gay. Cotton (1992) noted that convictions of gay-bashers are few and far between. In 1991, 600 cases of gay-bashing were followed through the New York City courts: Only two resulted in convictions.

The gay or bisexual man who is the victim of a hate crime may be unwilling to report the attack, for fear of secondary victimization. In 1991, there were 146 reports of physical assault of lesbian, gay, or bisexual people by police officers in New York City. If the victim ends up in a hospital, he may face other forms of secondary victimization, such as insensitive treatment, being assumed heterosexual and the victim of random violence (which may force a disclosure), lack of belief that the crime was antigay, fear of publicity (more closeted gay and bisexual men may fear that their names will be printed in the paper), and harassment and/or discrimination from hospital staff.

When the hate crime involves a sexual assault, the gay or bisexual male victim faces other potential problems. Hospital staff may not believe that a man can be raped, or they may believe that all gay/bisexual men want to be raped, or that he brought it on himself. Most sexual assaults of gay and bisexual men are by heterosexual men, using sexual assault as a brutal means of asserting power and humiliation on the victim. Hickson et al. (1994) reported the case of a man who was raped (forced anal intercourse) by six work colleagues after finding out he was gay. The victim was subsequently fired from his job (another example of secondary victimization).

Many gay and bisexual men are victims of some type of physical or sexual assault in their lifetimes. Berrill (1992) summarized the findings of several studies and found that gay and bisexual men experienced verbal abuse (64%-77%) and physical attacks (6%-35%) more often than lesbians. Partly this is due to gay and bisexual men being more visible in public life, especially in gay-identified areas such as bars or gay neighborhoods. Men are more likely to be out late at night than women. Lesbian, gay, and bisexual people of color are especially vulnerable to attack and harassment.

In one gay-bashing episode, a gay man met two young men in a gay bar. They were very friendly and invited him to accompany them to a party. But instead of going to a party, they drove him to a remote, deserted park:

They forced me at knife point to strip. They beat me. . . . They threatened to castrate me. They threatened to emasculate me. They called me "Queer," "Faggot." One of them urinated on me. They threatened me with sodomy. . . . Finally, I think I probably was close to passing out. . . . They relaxed a little bit. They stopped kicking me around for a few minutes while they talked. One of them said to the other one, "Let's finish him off and get out of here." The one holding the knife raised the knife over his head and swung it at my throat. I reached up and grabbed the blade of the knife to avoid it going through my throat and managed to roll my body into his legs. He fell across me. I managed to get out from under him and I ran for my life. . . . The boys were seniors at St. John's College High School. . . . I spent five days in the hospital. . . . The boys were at school the next day. That is how long they stayed in police custody. . . . Judge Nunzio put off sentencing at the convenience of the boy's high school graduation. . . . he proceeded to give the boys unsupervised probation for a period of three years. . . . [one of the boy's parents] comment on leaving the room was that he certainly wasn't going to pay some faggot for getting his son in trouble. (Hassel, 1992, pp. 144-146)

As Herek (1992) noted, "Anti-gay violence is a logical, albeit extreme, extension of the heterosexism that pervades American society" (p. 89). Until all states protect people from discrimination and violence based on sexual identity, until churches stop preaching hatred from their pulpits, until the legal system punishes the perpetrators of antigay violence, lesbian, gay, and bisexual people will continue to live in fear.

Potential Consequences of Internalized Homophobia

Internalized homophobia plagues many gay and bisexual men. They apply negative stereotypes to themselves or other gay people along a continuum from mild self-doubts or guilt to reluctance to be seen with openly gay people, to extreme self-hatred and self-destructive behavior. This negative conditioning runs deep, and few lesbian, gay, and bisexual people can fully escape its effects. While overcoming internalized homophobia takes considerable effort and time, the coming out process can help lesbian, gay, and bisexual people start to unlearn stereotypes and begin to see themselves and other lesbian, gay, and bisexual people as unique individuals. Some reach a level of self-acceptance and pride in themselves, but others remain mired in earlier, more negative stages, or lack positive role models and are at risk for the consequences of internalized homophobia: depression and suicide, substance abuse, altered body image (see Chapter 6), and relationship problems including domestic violence (see Chapter 4). These problems can be exacerbated by societal stigma, and need to be carefully studied (Rothblum, 1994).

Depression and Suicide.   Like lesbians and bisexual women, gay and bisexual men are at higher risk for suicide attempts and depression than the general population. Bell and Weinberg (1978) found that African American gay men were 12 times more likely and European American gay men were 3 times more likely than the general population of men in the United States to think about or attempt suicide. Most attempts occurred during the adolescent years.

Cochran and Mays (1994) studied a national sample of 829 homosexually active African American men, of whom 80% identified themselves as gay, 14% as bisexual, and 5% as neither, but currently sexually active with men. The sample had a mean age of 33.4. The questionnaire included an item about HIV status, and by self-report, 36% were HIV negative as of their last testing, 36% did not know their HIV status, and 29% were HIV positive. Of the 237 men who were HIV positive, 120 were symptomatic of AIDS. Table 8.1 shows the depression scores of the men in this sample compared with mostly White gay men and mostly heterosexual African American men. The rates of probable clinical depression were very high, especially in the HIV-positive men, but even those who were HIV negative had higher rates of depression than samples of White gay men or heterosexual African American men. Suicidal thoughts were fairly common, and 5% of the symptomatic HIV-positive men reported that suicidal thoughts were their most upsetting life problem. Men who were HIV negative experienced as much depression as HIV-positive asymptomatic men.

Depression is an understandable reaction to societal rejection and discrimination, and internalized homophobia and internalized racism. Greene (1994) noted:

> *Ethnic minority gay men and lesbians exist as minorities within minorities with the multiple levels of oppression and discrimination that accompanies such status. They bear the additional task of integrating two major aspects of their identity when both are conspicuously devalued; their sexual orientation*

TABLE 8.1. Studies of Depression Using the Center for Epidemiologic Studies-Depression (CES-D) Scale with Various Populations

Sample	CES-D Mean Score	Percentage with Scores > 15*
Men in general	7.1	
Gay men (> 90% White)	9.9	
African American men (mostly heterosexual)	9.8	23
African American Gay/Bisexual men		
Symptomatic HIV+	16.7	47
Asymptomatic HIV+	12.8	32
HIV negative	12.7	34
HIV status unknown	11.4	26

*A score of greater than 15 indicates probable clinical depression.
Note. Adapted from Cochran and Mays (1994).

may be devalued by those closest to them. . . . Regardless of the specific ethnic group to which they belong, they must manage the dominant culture's racism, sexism, and its heterosexism. They must also manage the sexism, heterosexism, and internalized racism of their own ethnic group. For most gays and lesbians of ethnic minority groups, their ties to their ethnic communities are of great practical and emotional significance. They may be important havens against racism, as well as important sources of support. The homophobia in these communities makes gay and lesbian members more vulnerable and perhaps more inclined to remain closeted, and hence, invisible within their ethnic communities. (Greene, 1994, p. 248)

Health care providers need to recognize symptoms of depression in their patients/clients and know counseling sources that will be sensitive to issues of race and sexuality.

Domestic Violence: Sexual Abuse by Partners.   Waterman, Dawson, and Bologna (1989) found that 12% of the men in their sample of 24 gay men had been sexually assaulted by a recent or current partner. Hickson et al. (1994) interviewed 930 homosexually active men and found that 28% had been subjected to nonconsensual sex at some time in their lives, and 5% had been molested by their regular sexual partner. The authors noted:

Characterizing male rape as a crime of violence, power, and control may trivialize the emotional trauma suffered by men who are raped by casual sex partners. It may also place them in a similar position as many women who have been raped. Typical responses to reporting could be "You were asking for it," "What did you expect?" "You wanted it or you wouldn't have gone with him in the first place," "You enjoyed it really." Fantasies of the sexually forceable man, the pleasure of "being taken," and the excitement of power-driven sex are very common in gay culture and pornography. All these collective sexual fantasies normalize sexual abuse and rape of gay men by gay men, providing motivation, justification, and normalization for the assault. (p. 293)

Nonconsensual sex among gay men and date rape among heterosexual women have striking similarities. The heterosexual "rape culture," which portrays women as always wanting sex and wanting to be taken, is reproduced in much gay pornography. Sexual violence is not limited to male-female relationships, and victims of rape, regardless of their sex, often require support and sensitive care and counseling to deal with the trauma of the experience.

Substance Abuse.   Early studies with somewhat suspect methodologies reported a high prevalence of alcohol abuse or dependence among gay men, at least those in urban areas, who have been the most studied (Fifield, 1975; Icard & Traunstein, 1987; Lohrenz, Connelly, Coyne, & Spare, 1978). More recent work, however, is beginning to show somewhat different patterns. For example, Stall and Wiley (1988) found that 75% of the gay men in their sample were frequent drinkers, but only 19% were frequent and heavy drinkers, and only some of those could be classified as alcohol dependent. Thus, heavy drinking and/or frequent drinking, but not necessarily alcohol dependence could typify many gay and bisexual men.

McKirnan and Peterson (1989a) surveyed 2,652 gay and bisexual men from Chicago about their alcohol and drug use. They had a mean age of 35, and 88% were European American, 7% were African American, and 3% were Latino. As a group, they were highly educated. Table 8.2 shows the rates of alcohol dependency and marijuana and cocaine use in this sample compared with the general population of men. As men in the general population age, they decrease their alcohol intake, but gay and bisexual men in this sample continued to have heavier drinking even at later ages. However, if you compare the general population rates for abstinence from alcohol (14%), more lesbian, gay, and bisexual people abstain (29%). Rates of heavy drinking were 14% for the general population and 15% for the lesbian, gay, and bisexual sample. The major difference was in the rate of moderate drinkers: 57% of the general population, but 71% of the lesbian, gay, and bisexual sample, reported moderate levels of alcohol intake.

Weinberg (1994) studied the role that alcohol plays in the lives of gay men and gay communities. He interviewed 46 urban gay men, aged 21-68 (mean age, 29), obtained through a newspaper ad, members of a men's support group, and friends of previous respondents (snowball technique); most were European American. By drinking patterns, 6 men were abstainers and recovering alcoholics, 4 were self-identified alcoholics but were still drinking, and the rest were moderately heavy to

TABLE 8.2.   Rates of Alcohol Dependency, Marijuana, and Cocaine Use among Gay and Bisexual Men and Men in the General Population, by Age Group

Age	General Population: Men (%)	Gay and Bisexual Men (%)
Alcohol Dependency		
18–25	29	26
26–30	25	25
31–40	16	24
41–60	7	19
Lifetime Use: Marijuana		
18–25	68	79
26–34	65	83
35+	17	67
Frequent Use: Marijuana		
18–25	23	16
26–34	11	16
35+	2	8
Lifetime Use: Cocaine		
18–25	35	52
26–34	26	56
35+	7	26
Frequent Use: Cocaine		
18–25	3	3
26–34	1	4
35+	0.1	0.5

Note. Adapted from McKirnan and Peterson (1989a).

heavy drinkers. The sample is not necessarily representative of the gay and bisexual men's community, but since Weinberg was not attempting to find the incidence of drinking, this is not a major concern. Instead, the author collected rich data about the drinking contexts of gay men. He noted that friendships play a more central role in the lives of lesbian, gay, and bisexual people, who may or may not have family or other community support. Thus, friends serve as role models and social support in an often oppressive world. Weinberg explored the role of drinking within friendship networks and found that people within a friendship network generally have the same patterns of drinking. Drinking is often part of gay men's friendship socializing, and the men in this study rarely drank alone. As one respondent put it:

> *Social life is really limited in the gay world to where, when you go to someplace socially in public, you don't really have a*

choice. There's always alcohol there and that's what everyone is
partaking of. I suppose I wouldn't have to, but it just becomes a
way of life after awhile. I would say that 90% of gay people . . .
I know who have a social life drink three or four days a week.
(Weinberg, 1994, p. 20)

The setting for drinking was most often gay bars (41% did most of
their drinking there), but alcohol was also a central part of private parties and dinner parties in these men's friendship circles. The amount of
drinking in bars was a variable that distinguished gay men from heterosexual men—gay men do much more of their drinking in bars. While
heterosexual men often drink heavily in their adolescent and young
adult years and often frequent bars, their drinking tends to decrease
along with declining bar attendance as they age. Gay men tend to maintain higher levels of drinking and bar attendance. The importance of gay
bars for gay and bisexual men cannot be discounted. Hooker (1967)
noted that gay bars "serve as induction and training centers for the community" (p. 178). The gay bar is a refuge from the homophobic world—
it is where friends gather and where lovers meet. The negative impact of
bars as a social phenomenon is its pattern of heavy drinking:

If I go to a bar, it's nearly impossible not to drink. Well, I have
gone to bars and haven't drunk, but also, it's a situation
around you. . . . I don't have as good a time because everyone's
drunk and I think I have to be. It's a matter of—I don't think its
conforming with them, but I think it's a situation of the setting,
too. (Weinberg, 1994, p. 41)

Peer pressure to drink can be strong in gay bars (as in other bars), and
alcohol is sometimes used for its disinhibitory effects—giving the person "courage" to ask someone to dance or to approach a potential sexual
partner. However, alcohol also impairs judgment in sexual situations.
The role of alcohol in unsafe sexual experiences is not entirely clear.
The commonsense argument is that people under the influence of alcohol (or other drugs) are less likely to take precautions (Molgaard,
NaKamwa, Hovell, & Elder, 1988; Nardi, 1991; Ruefli, Yu, & Barton,
1992). There is also evidence that prolonged heavy drinking weakens
the immune system, making the person more susceptible to viruses including HIV.

Weinberg (1994) also found that drinking was part of couple relationships for many gay men, and not just part of a singles bar scene.

Many of his respondents thought that alcohol was a part of an "elegant" lifestyle—they had drinks upon arriving home after work, drinks with dinner, and maybe a "nightcap" later on. Drinking was a central part of entertaining, so that even men whose bar attendance declined maintained high levels of alcohol intake. Heavy drinking within a couple's relationship often caused conflicts, but many found it hard to quit or reduce drinking if their partner (and their friends) drank heavily.

A number of explanations for the high rates of drinking among gay and bisexual men have been proposed. Some have suggested that drinking is in response to alienation—feeling left out of a mainstream society; others suggest that drinking is one means of coping with oppression and the stress of identity management; yet others point to the central role of gay bars and the lack of nondrinking alternatives for social life. Weinberg found no evidence for alienation, but instead offered the Reference Group theory: "People drink because their friends drink, and they regulate their drinking in terms of the usually unstated norms of their group" (p. 146). This theory includes the idea of the bar as the main social institution of the gay community—the "unstated norms" of the community these men lived in included bar attendance and drinking.

Drug use among gay and bisexual men also appears to exceed rates of the general population of men, and it does not show the decline with age as is expected. McKirnan and Peterson's study included questions about lifetime and current use of marijuana and cocaine (see Table 8.2), and suggested that the main differences were in lifetime use—frequent use was not very different from that of the general population.

Skinner (1994) examined the rates of a range of licit and illicit substances in 265 gay men with a mean age of 37. The vast majority (94%) were White. Table 8.3 shows these findings by age group, and reports only on recent use. The drugs of highest use were alcohol, cigarettes, marijuana, and inhalants (particularly amyl nitrate or "poppers"). Skinner found that higher education was associated with lower marijuana and cigarette use, but living in an urban area was associated with increased smoking. Higher income, urban living, and being in a close relationship resulted in increased alcohol use.

McKirnan and Peterson (1989b) also looked at predicters of alcohol and drug use and found that degree of outness was associated with frequent alcohol use, frequency of intoxication, alcohol problems, marijuana and cocaine use, and drug problems for their male respondents.

TABLE 8.3. Substance Use by Gay and Bisexual Men in Month prior to Survey

Drug	Age		
	18–25 (%)	26–34 (%)	35+ (%)
Marijuana	38	16	15
Cocaine	4	2	2
Crack	0	0	0
Inhalants	17	14	18
Hallucinogens	8	0	8
Heroin	0	0	0
Stimulants	22	4	2
Sedatives	4	0	2
Tranquilizers	0	2	2
Analgesics	3	3	1
Psychotherapeutics	29	6	3
Alcohol	83	81	70
Cigarettes	58	26	35

Note. Adapted from Skinner (1994).

Role status (mostly related to occupational roles) had the same effects as outness. Relationship status did not predict any substance use variables, nor did conflict about sexual orientation predict alcohol or drug use. Among vulnerable men (those with cultural values and attitudes related to alcohol as a tension reducer and expectations that alcohol and bar life would improve the quality of their lives), discrimination due to sexual orientation was related to higher alcohol and drug use. This was not found for low vulnerable men or women. Some men reported use of alcohol and drugs to cope with personal stress (23% used alcohol and 10% used drugs as a coping mechanism).

Gay and bisexual men with alcohol or drug problems, like lesbians and bisexual women, often encounter discrimination or harassment in treatment centers. Hellman, Stanton, Lee, Tytun, and Vachon (1989) surveyed staff and administrators from 36 alcohol treatment agencies in New York City. The 164 respondents (64 male and 94 female) fell mostly in the 35–44 age group; 47% were European American, 31% were African American, 17% were Latino, and 4% were Asian American. Over 80% had college degrees, and most had little or no training about homosexual clients (71%). However, the majority said that 1%–25% of their clients in the past year were homosexual (76%). A significant number of

the staff members asked about sexual orientation of their clients in intake interviews (21% always and 22% most of the time), yet 33% never or
almost never did. Regarding treatment outcomes, 38% thought that homosexual clients had more difficulty achieving sobriety than heterosexual clients, and 44% thought they had the same level of difficulty. Nearly
half of the staff thought it would be helpful to have openly gay staff
(10% of respondents were lesbian, gay, or bisexual themselves), although
only 43% of the respondents said that their agency had gay staff members. Treatment programs rarely had any special groups or programs for
homosexual clients (only 6%).

GAY AND BISEXUAL MEN'S PHYSICAL HEALTH

Other than for the higher rates of HIV/AIDS, gay and bisexual men
seem to be more similar to heterosexual men in physical health ailments than different. Gay and bisexual men may suffer more stress-
related disorders due to the societal stigma of homosexuality, but there
is no empirical support of this supposition. One way that gay and bisexual men do differ, as a group, is in the rate of sexually transmitted
infections and medical conditions related to sexual activity.

Unsafe Sexual Experiences

A consistent difference between men and women in our society is their
attitudes about and engagement in casual sex—men have more positive
attitudes about it and are more likely to engage in casual sex. Because of
this gender difference in attitudes, men who have sex with other men
are much more likely to find willing partners for casual sex. This is not
to say that all gay and bisexual men constantly seek out casual sex, but
that, as a group, gay and bisexual men have more sex than lesbian and bisexual women and heterosexual couples (Weinberg, Williams, & Pryor,
1994). The higher the rate of sexual activity, particularly if it is with
more than one partner, the higher the risk for all types of sexually transmitted infections and related medical illnesses. O'Neill and Shalit (1992)
reviewed a wide range of conditions for which the sexually active gay or
bisexual man should routinely be evaluated. Table 8.4 lists some of the
possible conditions.

TABLE 8.4. Sexually Transmitted Diseases and Related Medical Conditions Often Found in Sexually Active Gay and Bisexual Men

Human papillomavirus
Anogenital warts
Anal cancer (rare)
Proctitis
Enteritis
Gonorrhea
Syphilis
Hepatitis
Rectal or anal trauma

Note. Adapted from O'Neill and Shalit (1992).

O'Neill and Shalit recommended that sexually active gay and bisexual men have annual digital rectal exams to screen for anal cancer, regardless of their age (the American Cancer Society recommends annual exams only for men over 40). They also noted that any sexually transmitted infection or condition represents possible exposure to HIV, and that STIs have been implicated as cofactors in HIV transmission.

Proctitis can be caused by infectious agents (e.g., herpes simplex virus, chalmydia) or noninfectious factors (e.g., trauma or allergic reactions to lubricants). Since proctitis can exist with few or no symptoms, the authors recommend annual anoscopy as well. O'Neill and Shalit also noted that symptoms of pharyngitis can be an early sign of HIV infection and/or can be due to an oral gonococcal infection. Hepatitis (all varieties) can be sexually transmitted and thus should be considered in the annual exam. Anal trauma is not common in gay and bisexual men, but it can occur when sex was not consensual, when there is a lack of proper lubrication, or when the patient was under the influence of a substance that dulled pain perception. Rectal foreign bodies are sometimes encountered, often long after the fact because the patient is too embarrassed to seek help. Surgical intervention may be required to remove foreign bodies.

The higher incidence of these medical complications of high sexual activity highlight the need for safer-sex discussions. Many health care providers are uncomfortable talking to clients or patients about specific sexual behaviors. The preceding problems, however, as well as HIV, show the need for explicit sex education. Since very few of us received this kind of education in high school, or even in college, the burden often falls on us as health care providers to seek out knowledge and experience in sex education. A wide variety of health care professionals need this knowledge—anyone who works in obstetrics and gynecology, STD clinics, family practice settings, free medical clinics, student health, high schools, adolescent medicine, or any community health agency. Table 8.5 lists some common sexual practices of gay and bisexual men from relatively safe to unsafe. These behaviors can be found in any sexual encounter—with heterosexual, lesbian, gay, or bisexual people, and the risks apply for HIV as well as other sexually transmitted infections.

TABLE 8.5. Gay and Bisexual Male Sexual Behaviors: Lowest to Highest Theoretical Risk

Low Risk	Abstinence
	Solo masturbation
	Dry kissing
	Wet kissing
	Mutual masturbation, only external touching
	Frottage (rubbing against a person for sexual pleasure)
	Fellatio without a condom, but without putting the head of the penis inside the mouth
Medium	Fellatio to orgasm with a condom
	Fellatio without a condom, putting the head of the penis in the mouth, but withdrawing before ejaculation
	Fellatio without a condom with ejaculation in the mouth
	Anal intercourse with a condom, lubricant, and withdrawal prior to ejaculation
	Anal intercourse with a condom, lubricant, spermicide, with ejaculation
	Fisting (Brachioproctic activity—inserting a fist into the rectum)
	Anal intercourse with a condom and withdrawal before ejaculation
High Risk	Anal intercourse without a condom and with internal ejaculation

Note. Adapted from Stine (1995).

HIV/AIDS

> *It finally happened. After years of seeing friends, close and distant, buried, my news came. Or as so many PWA's (Persons with AIDS) can attest, "the news" finally came. At the age of 35, having lived through the "do as you please, have who you want, 70s," it was not if I get AIDS, but when. . . . I'm shocked, I'm scared. I'm numb. But at the same time, its not so horrible as the constant fear of AIDS. It's finally here. Like so many PWAs, I'm really able to say that the diagnosis isn't as bad as the anxiety. . . . Now more than ever, all the fiery sermons I had ever preached will now, as a preacher with AIDS, have to keep me alive. (Angel, 1993, pp. 47–48)*

This section will briefly review some issues that gay and bisexual men with AIDS may face. First, reviewing the history of HIV/AIDS will help place it in perspective. Table 8.6 provides a timeline of AIDS events in the United States. AIDS has had a very different course in Africa, where it is a primarily heterosexual disease that afflicts more women than men. In the United States and other Western countries, however, HIV/AIDS has disproportionately affected gay and bisexual men. In 1994, 43% of the new cases of AIDS were reportedly due to male-male sexual contact, compared with 27% of the cases due to needle sharing and 10% due to heterosexual sexual contact. About 5% of the cases were in gay or bisexual men who were also IV drug users (MMWR, February 3, 1995). AIDS has disproportionately affected African American and Latino men, a significant number of whom are also gay or bisexual. Peterson (1995) noted that among African American men who are HIV positive, 38% of the cases are attributed to IV drug use and 36% to homosexual sexual activity. More African American and Latino HIV positive men (41% and 31% respectively) report bisexual activity than European American men (21%). Among Latino men, terms like gay and bisexual have less meaning. Instead they may divide men into *activos* (the active or inserter role in sex) versus *pasivos* (the passive or receptive partner). Activos generally do not consider themselves gay or bisexual, and do not perceive themselves to be at risk for HIV (Carballo-Diéguez, 1995).

In Chapter 5, I reviewed several studies about health care provider attitudes, including a few that focused on the intersection between

TABLE 8.6. HIV/AIDS Timeline

Date	Event
1981	First reports of immune system failures and rare cancers in gay men in the medical literature: called GRID (Gay Related Immune Disease)
1982	Same symptoms reported in hemophiliacs; disease renamed AIDS
1983	First cases reported in heterosexuals via sexual contact (2 women who were partners of IV drug users)
1983	Luc Montanier and team in France isolate virus
1984	Robert Gallo and team in United States isolate virus
1985	First test to detect HIV antibodies approved for use
1985	Rock Hudson dies of AIDS, beginning public response to disease
1987	AZT (Zidovudine) becomes first drug approved for treatment of AIDS
1990	Ryan White, 18-year-old hemophiliac AIDS educator dies of AIDS
1991	Magic Johnson announces he is HIV positive; AIDS education efforts increase
1992	Second strain of AIDS identified (HIV-2); mostly in Africa
1993	CDC changes the definition of AIDS to one based on T-cell counts
1994	Largest number of new cases yet reported (over 103,000 adults and adolescents and 900 children)
1995	Over 300,000 adults and 3,400 children have died of AIDS; AIDS becomes leading cause of death among young men.

Note. Adapted from Stine (1995).

attitudes about homosexuality and bisexuality and attitudes about AIDS. In this chapter, I will review a few more studies and explore the implications of their findings. Then I will discuss issues related to treatment and AIDS prevention in gay and bisexual men.

Health Care Provider Attitudes about AIDS

Early in the AIDS epidemic, Blumenfield et al. surveyed about 300 nurses in two consecutive years—1983 and 1984 (Blumenfield, Smith, Milazzo, Seropian, & Wormser, 1987). These nurses indicated that their family or friends worried about their working with AIDS patients

(35%-81%), and that AIDS had made them more fearful of caring for male patients in general (22%-65%) and male homosexual patients specifically (14%-54%). Overall, they indicated more fear of working with patients who had AIDS than working with patients who had infectious hepatitis. Awareness of AIDS had made these nurses more concerned about working with gay male patients than they had been in the past (43% were more concerned in 1983, but only 25% were more concerned in 1984). Many nurses believed that pregnant staff should not care for AIDS patients (85%-89%). A significant number said that they would ask for a transfer if they had to work with AIDS patients on a regular basis, although the percentage dropped from 50% in 1983 to 39% in 1984, indicating that better AIDS education had reduced some of the negative attitudes.

Scherer, Haughey, and Wu (1989) surveyed 581 nurses randomly selected from all the RNs in a particular county in New York State. Most (95%) were female, and the sample had a mean age of 38. Half of the sample reported that they were fearful of contracting AIDS from a patient, and 56% said that getting AIDS from a patient was their major concern. Nearly half also worried about putting their families at risk, and 35% reported that caring for patients with AIDS would affect their relationships with significant others. Most believed that nurses should be assigned to care for AIDS patients only on a voluntary basis (61%), and 47% said they had a right to refuse to care for a PWA. Although most of the nurses in the sample acknowledged that dying patients need nursing support (93%), a significant number were uncomfortable with dying patients (24%). The authors also measured attitudes about homosexuality, and found that the majority of nurses were more sympathetic toward patients who had acquired HIV from a blood transfusion than from homosexual sex. Over half felt that they would not be comfortable establishing a therapeutic relationship with a homosexual patient (55%). Most believed, however, that the partners of homosexual patients deserve the same courtesy and respect as partners of heterosexual patients. Factors that influenced the nurses' attitudes included (1) religion (nurses with no religious beliefs were less fearful of contracting AIDS and had more positive attitudes about homosexuality); (2) being a parent (nurses without children were also less fearful and more positive); and (3) experience (working with patients with AIDS led to less fear and concern about caring for other AIDS patients but did not affect attitudes about homosexuality).

Haring and Lind (1992) surveyed 81 dental hygiene students about AIDS care. Each student read a vignette (taken from the research of Kelly et al. 1987, 1988) about a gay man with AIDS, a heterosexual man with AIDS, a gay man with leukemia, or a heterosexual man with leukemia. The students in this study evaluated the men with AIDS differently from the men with leukemia, but their ratings did not differ by sexuality. Patients with AIDS were rated as more responsible for their illness, as deserving of what happened to them, as more dangerous to others, and as more deserving to lose their jobs. Students indicated that they would not want even casual contact with the person with AIDS and would be unwilling to work in the same office or maintain a past friendship with the person.

Cole and Slocumb (1993) sent questionnaires to 357 nurses in New England. The sample was 96% female and 70% were in the 31–50 age range. Nearly all of these nurses (94%) had cared for a patient with AIDS. Most of them (70%) did not consider themselves, their friends, or their family members to be at risk for HIV. In this study, the authors chose to study attitudes about the modes of transmission (sex with men, sex with women, needle sharing, blood transfusion). In all cases, the nurses were to rate "a male who acquired AIDS through . . . (one of the four modes of transmission) according to semantic differential scales, such as good/bad, guilty/innocent, immoral/moral, and dangerous/safe. Nurses were more positive about male patients who acquired AIDS through blood transfusions than other modes and were most negative about needle sharing and sex with men. The authors noted that nurses' negative attitudes about some (or most) AIDS patients not only affect patient care adversely, but also lead to lower work productivity and burnout. Thus, such attitudes should be a major area of concern for educators and administrators.

Harrison, Fisilier, and Worley (1994) administered an attitude survey to 225 nurses, in an attempt to find a brief, but psychometrically sound instrument for use in the clinical setting. They found that their measure was reliable (coefficient alpha of .69 to .92), and that it had three factors. Factor 1 related to conservative views about religion, family, politics, and homosexuality; Factor 2 assessed willingness to provide care; and Factor 3 measured feelings of sympathy toward homosexuals and IV drug users since the AIDS epidemic started. The importance of this research is that nurses' attitudes are based not only on factual knowledge about AIDS, but also on underlying conservative views. Thus, providing education alone will not change negative attitudes in all health care providers.

Although we have only anecdotal information about the ways that negative attitudes and fears of AIDS can manifest in health care providers' behaviors, these attitudes likely manifest in some of the same ways as homophobia—as a continuum from mild discomfort to avoidance to violence. However, the specter of contagion gives AIDS an added dimension. Some people with AIDS have reported being treated with extreme precautions, even in situations where there is no risk.

Herek and Glunt (1988) discussed the interactions of homophobia and a phenomenon they labeled "AIDS-related stigma." This concept combines societal fears of death and dying with fears of contracting a terminal illness. Thus, even health care providers who are not homophobic may have difficulty caring for patients with AIDS. Additionally, AIDS is one of the few diseases whereby some health care providers assign blame, and distinguish among "guilty" versus "innocent" victims.

Prevention of HIV

One friend told me that there were many nights he went to bed wishing he were positive, that the guilt he felt about being healthy while his lover and friends were either positive or dying was unbearable. Here he was, deeply involved in the HIV crisis, but an unacknowledged participant—unacknowledged even to himself. His life is thoroughly affected, but somehow his situation remains somewhat invalidated by being HIV negative. (Slocum, 1993, p. 84)

Once I was settled in the States, the phone started ringing. It was L.A., or Frisco, or N.Y. informing me that someone had died or someone was sick. It got so bad that each time the phone rang, I would start shaking uncontrollably, feel light-headed and break out in a cold sweat. (Dunn, 1993, p. 64)

These quotes give some small indication of what it is like to be a gay or bisexual man living in the AIDS epidemic. Dean (1995) found that 98% of homosexual respondents reported feeling under stress in 1994—compared with 89% of heterosexuals. The anxieties about becoming HIV positive appear to be no less than the guilt about being healthy—fears of HIV/AIDS may be incapacitating for some. It is somewhat hard for people to believe that the AIDS epidemic is continuing, despite what we know about transmission. Why aren't all gay and bisexual men using condoms and reducing their risks in every way possible? Prevention of any unhealthy behavior is difficult. Think about smoking. We have known about the health hazards of smoking for a long time, yet a significant number of people continue to smoke. Why? What about drinking or heroin use or lack of exercise?

Sandfort (1995) suggested that negative societal attitudes about homosexuality and bisexuality have interfered with prevention activities in several ways. First, at the institutional level, homophobia has affected the governmental response to HIV. Moral and religious attitudes, rather than science, influenced public health decisions, and the epidemic was allowed to progress unchecked much longer than it should have. Second, some authors suggest that internalized homophobia affects prevention at the individual level, although the data are certainly not completely clear on this count. Some studies have found that men with internalized homophobia are more likely to engage in high-risk sexual activities (Prieur, 1990), yet many others have found no link between internalized homophobia and unsafe sex (Hayes, Kegeles, & Coates, 1990; Sandfort, 1995; Shidlo, 1994). In fact, in some of these studies, gay men with more social support and more gay friends were *more likely* to engage in high-risk sex. Likewise, the relationship between safer sex and "outness" is not clear—some studies have found no relationship (Hays, Kegeles, & Coates, 1990), whereas some have found that the more out the man is, the higher the likelihood of engaging in casual sex (Connell et al., 1990). Being involved with the gay community has been identified as a risk factor for unsafe sex in some studies (Sandfort, 1995) and a protective factor in others (Kippax et al., 1992). Being depressed may be related to unsafe sex (Ekstrand & Coates, 1990), or not (Vincke, Bolton, Mak, & Blank, 1993). Herek and Glunt (1995) suggested that gay community and individual psychological variables related to being gay or bisexual are not direct predictors of sexual risk, but can mediate sexual risk through attitudes about risk reduction. They also noted that psychological factors, such as accepting one's own sexuality and having support in gay communities, lead to better mental health, which allows for better coping with the stresses of HIV/AIDS. Herek and Glunt suggested that the conflicting findings about risk factors for unsafe sex are the result of considering gay and bisexual men to be a monolithic group—instead, we need to consider them as existing in various subgroups that vary by sexual identity, age, race, basic personality styles, and so on.

In a longitudinal study of gay and bisexual men, Ostrow, Beltran, and Joseph (1994) summarized data from over 1,000 volunteers who entered the study in 1984. They examined rates of receptive anal sex (RAS), since it is the sexual activity associated with the highest risk for transmission of HIV. As a group, the rates of unprotected RAS declined over the study period, from about 50% in 1984 to less than 30% in 1989-1990. Among individuals, however, only about 10%-15% of those men who reported unprotected RAS at the first visit had adopted consistent condom use or restricted their unprotected RAS to a single partner. Many initially chose to abstain from RAS, but at least 33% of the abstainers "relapsed" each year. Declines in alcohol and drug use were also reported over the years, and less than 1% reported any needle drug use. A subset of 177 men requested to know their HIV status. Those who reported increased risk taking after learning their HIV status were different on psychological profiles from men who maintained low risk behaviors or decreased their risk taking after learning their HIV status. The increased risk takers were characterized by greater denial and fatalism, lower social support, lower feelings of validation, greater feelings of social conflict and isolation, greater depression, and lower income and education. As Herek and Glunt had suggested, these authors found different psychological subgroups within the larger sample.

These studies provide a muddled picture for those interested in HIV prevention activities—if there is no clear profile of the person who is likely to engage in high-risk behavior, who should be targeted for prevention education and how should this education be done? The challenge lies ahead of us. HIV/AIDS can be prevented, but only when health care providers and educators become comfortable talking about sex in explicit terms. Thus far, what passes for "sex education" and "safe-sex messages" are often too vague to be helpful. We must be explicit about sexual activities (not sexual identity groups), and teach all of our clients how to protect themselves. We should not forget to support and encourage the "worried well" and the healthy caretakers of loved ones with AIDS—the epidemic has taken a tremendous toll on these caretakers as they watch their loved ones sicken and die.

Conclusion

In the 1990s, gay and bisexual men's mental and health problems primarily center around HIV/AIDS and other sexually transmitted infections. Health care providers need further education to prepare them to be sex educators for their clients, and they need to know how to adapt safe-sex education for audiences that differ by sexual identity, age, race, and other variables. In a time when sex can kill, the benefits of frank discussion about sexuality in our society cannot be underestimated.

EXERCISE: AIDS IN REAL LIFE

Imagine that your current or most recent sexual partner has just told you that she/he is HIV positive. What would be your initial reaction? Would it be anger, fear, despair, concern about your own HIV status? What would be the first questions you would ask this partner? Would it matter how she/he got the virus? Why? Do you think you would stay in the relationship? If so, how would your families react? What about your friends? Could you count on your best friend to support you in this crisis? Reactions to HIV/AIDS are complex and sometimes illogical. How can you help your clients grapple with these and other questions that will arise from an HIV or AIDS diagnosis?

CHAPTER NINE

Making Health Care Safe and Inclusive

WHEREAS THE HOMOSEXUAL PATIENT MAY merely be avoided by hospital staff, the loved one often incurs their outright hostility, for they see him [sic] as interfering where he has no business. The loved one finds himself unable to obtain information about the patient or to participate in decisions that relate to his care. At a time when his energy should be channeled into care and concern for someone he loves, it must be expended instead on bureaucratic hassles in dealing with the fact that he is not recognized as having a legitimate role to play in the situation, or coping with the devaluation of the relationship. . . . To endure a hospital stay may be one of the most bitter and unpleasant of any of the oppressive experiences that homosexual persons are subject to daily. (Lawrence, 1975, pp. 307-308)

Before lesbian, gay, and bisexual people can receive high-quality health care on a regular basis, major changes are needed at three levels: the personal or individual health care provider, the institutional (health care systems, agencies, or organizations), and the societal (including national health care policy). These three areas overlap to a great extent, and societal changes might influence personal beliefs, changes in personal beliefs can have impact on health care institutions, and so on. For the sake of clarity, I will discuss each one separately, but keep in mind their interrelatedness. I will begin with a brief consideration of societal changes, then focus much of the chapter on the changes needed in health care institutions and individual health care providers.

SOCIETY AND THE HEALTHY HOMOSEXUAL

I borrowed the title of this section from a book by George Weinberg, originally written in 1972 and reprinted in 1991. He proposed that the major barrier that lesbian, gay, and bisexual people faced in the world was the negative attitudes of others close to them, and of society as a whole. In the absence of these negative attitudes, lesbian, gay, and bisexual people would be free to achieve their full human potential. Some would continue to have difficulty adjusting to the stresses of daily life and to have psychological and physical health problems, just as some heterosexuals suffer from depression, anxiety, or ulcers. However, sexual identity would no longer be a barrier to achieving human potential or to acquiring adequate health care. This is a somewhat simplistic approach since individual attitudes are only one part of the problem—institutional heterosexism creates and maintains negative individual attitudes. The civil rights movement taught us that deeply ingrained attitudes are difficult to dislodge, and that institutions are resistant to change. Yet a world free of bias and prejudice should be a goal we work for.

Most heterosexual people are not aware of the power of societal attitudes to adversely affect lesbian, gay, and bisexual people's lives. Some heterosexuals have been influenced by the very visible hate campaigns launched by a few Radical Right groups that declared that homosexuals wanted "special privileges" or that the "gay agenda" was threatening to take over the country. In reality, the "special privileges" that lesbian, gay, and bisexual people want are the basic human rights automatically afforded to heterosexuals such as equal access to educational opportunities, jobs, housing, and freedom from harassment and discrimination based solely on sexual identity. Suzanne Pharr (1988), in her book on homophobia, stated what lesbians want (and this could also apply to bisexuals and gay men):

> We want the elimination of homophobia. We are seeking equality. Equality is more than tolerance, compassion, understanding, acceptance, benevolence, for these still come from a place of implied superiority: favors granted to those less fortunate. These attitudes suggest that there is still something wrong, something not quite right that must be overlooked or seen beyond. The elimination of homophobia requires that

homosexual identity be viewed as viable and legitimate and as normal as heterosexual identity. It does not require tolerance; it requires an equal footing. Given the elimination of homophobia, sexual identity—whether homosexual, bi-sexual, or heterosexual—will not be seen as good or bad, but simply as what it is. (p. 45)

Since there is no unified lesbian, gay, and bisexual community with an "agenda," other than seeking respect, dignity, and equality, I would like to propose a lesbian, gay, and bisexual agenda for health care:

- Lesbian, gay, and bisexual people will be treated with respect, as human beings rather than as "sexual differences."
- Lesbian, gay, and bisexual families will be recognized as one of many legitimate forms of family, and they will be given all the rights and privileges of other families.
- Health care providers will not assume that sexual identity is a problem but will consider that, in our current homophobic society, it may be a factor in health and illness. In other words, sexual identity will be treated like other human characteristics such as age, race, and sex.
- Sexual identity will not be the reason to deny anyone the right to foster, adopt, conceive, gain, or retain custody of a child—parenting skills, the financial ability to support a child, and personality stability will be the deciding factors.
- No one will be asked to feel shame, guilt, or discomfort about her/his own sexual identity or that of a family member, friend, or coworker, thus disclosure of sexual identity will no longer be a stressful event.
- No one's sexual identity will be taken for granted—health care forms and interviews will routinely include questions about sexual identity, sexual history, and sexual behaviors, thus assuming a diversity of sexual experience instead of assuming a similarity of experience.

Achieving these goals will require procedural changes in health care systems as well as education of individual health care providers. For real acceptance of lesbian, gay, and bisexual people, however, education alone will not suffice. The negative stereotypes about lesbian, gay, and bisexual people are so entwined with religion, irrational prejudices, and fears that real change will require intensive personal reflection and challenging of those irrational beliefs. Changes in health care institutions (as well as other major societal institutions such as education, law, and the media would encourage this type of attitude readjustment). When policies and procedures are altered to stop discriminating against some group of people, they reveal negative attitudes for what they are; irrational prejudices.

HEALTH CARE INSTITUTIONS

Heterosexism is so deeply embedded in health care systems that it will require major efforts to ferret it out. At first glance, it may even be difficult to see the heterosexist bias, because antilesbian, gay, and bisexual sentiment is just taken for granted, or everyone is presumed to be heterosexual. Once you start to look for it, potential bias is everywhere—in hospital admission and health history forms, in the interview formats used by many health care providers that assume heterosexuality, in the educational pamphlets in clinics and waiting rooms, in the requirements for some procedures such as artificial insemination, in visiting hours policies, and in health care decision making and information sharing. Because of the pervasiveness of this bias, a multipronged approach is needed.

The general climate of the health care institution should first be evaluated (or if it is a very large institution, its individual units or departments). Is it overtly hostile to lesbian, gay, and bisexual clients/patients/employees, or is it characterized by benign neglect? Administrators need to determine the goal—do they want a tolerant environment or an accepting environment?

A tolerant environment would not hinder an employee's growth or chances for promotion, or overtly discriminate against lesbian, gay, or bisexual clients, but it would not encourage honesty and openness either. In a tolerant environment, lesbian, gay, and bisexual clients and employees would be asked to keep their sexual identities private and to assimilate into the heterosexist mold. Employees or clients/patients might be told, "Don't advertise your sexuality, and you will be just fine," or "It's okay to be lesbian, gay, or bisexual, but just don't talk about it at work." No accommodations would be made for difference, and people who are different by race or sexual identity might never be able to fit in. When people who cannot fit into the structure leave the institution, it tends to reinforce the stereotype that culturally different people cannot assimilate or are "too difficult" to work with. In reality, the institution made no effort to best utilize that person's talents or make her/him feel comfortable. The social atmosphere of the tolerant institution would necessarily be downplayed and the focus put on the work environment. The tolerant environment would probably operate from the equal treatment model—the policies and procedures would state that everyone is to be treated the same regardless of race, sex, sexual identity, and so on. The tolerant environment probably typifies most health care institutions today. The following scenario is a real-life example of the problems of a tolerant environment:

> *LaToya had worked as a respiratory therapist at the same hospital for five years before she came out to her boss and a few coworkers. She had been groomed for a promotion and was well-liked. When she came out to her supervisor, he had insisted that it would make no difference—that her work was valued. But the climate changed very quickly. Most people were still friendly to her face, but she was rarely invited to lunch or parties anymore. After she came out, her supervisor never mentioned the promotion again. Then one day, during a staff meeting, a new employee made a homophobic remark. Although several people looked uncomfortable and glanced at LaToya for her reaction, no one said anything. After a few months of this negative atmosphere, LaToya took another job.*

The accepting environment would consider client and employee diversity as good—administrators would be aware that their employees' varied skills and abilities enhanced the operation of the institution. Client/patient differences would also be valued and recognized in written forms, interviews, and the physical environment of the waiting room (by inclusion on posters, educational pamphlets, books, magazines, etc.). The environment would be flexible enough to accommodate difference; it would not have to push all people into the same pigeonholes. The social atmosphere would be considered an important facet of the institution, and honesty and openness would be encouraged. In this environment, LaToya would have received her promotion and the homophobic employee would have been quickly educated. LaToya's skills would not have been lost to the institution.

While the tolerant environment is easier to achieve because it requires fewer changes, it has many disadvantages. The lack of recognition of difference in employees and clients can lead to discriminatory care practices or unfair hiring/promotion practices. The need to keep sexual identity private (hidden) is a burden on both employees and clients and may lead to work burnout and loss of productivity, or loss of clients. An accepting environment is the preferable choice, so the rest of this section offers strategies for creating an accepting environment. Two main components of health care institutions can be modified to create a more accepting environment; education and training, and policies and procedures.

Education and Training

I challenge you to conduct a little research on your own. Review the major textbooks of your discipline or specialty area, and count the number of times that the words lesbian, gay, bisexual, or homosexual appear in the index. Look at the pages cited—does discussion of lesbian, gay, or bisexual issues fall under psychopathology, sexual deviance, or some other problem area? Are the references up to date? When I began the research for this book, I went to my health sciences library and typed "homosexuality" into the book reference computer program. I found only four books listed: Ed Bergler's *Homosexuality: Disease or Way of Life* (1962), a virulently negative diatribe against homosexuality which contains absolutely no empirical research, only the author's personal conjectures. I found Robert Kronemeyer's *Overcoming Homosexuality* (1980), which countered discussions of the need for compassionate care of the homosexual with statements that referred to homosexuals in derogatory slang terms and as "twisted" and "sick" individuals. Kronemeyer suggested that learning to express emotions, along with plenty of rest and good nutrition, could cure homosexuality. I found Richard von Krafft-Ebing's *Psychopathia Sexualis* (1886), a compendium of bizarre sexual case histories, and I found a 1970 human sexuality textbook for nurses with a chapter outlining homosexuality as a mental disorder. An uninformed student looking for answers about homosexuality would get a very biased and outmoded view from this selection of books, and would be seriously misled.

Survey your own health science library and if the selections are as abysmal as in my library, complain (I did). If the library were this deficient on some other topic, such as teen suicide or sudden infant death syndrome, we would be outraged. Forstein (1988) noted, "The failure to include in professional training programs the more recent psychologically sophisticated literature that debunks the old myths and stereotypes is the manifest expression of the profession's own homophobia, maintained in the face of scientific study to the contrary" (p. 34).

At this point in our history, some of the most up-to-date information about homosexuality and bisexuality for health care providers can be found in human sexuality textbooks, but even that is problematic. Total reliance on human sexuality texts implies that lesbian, gay, and bisexual issues are sexual issues only. As with heterosexual people, sexual behavior is only one small aspect of life for lesbian, gay, and bisexual people. In addition, most of these textbooks have separate chapters on lesbian, gay, and bisexual issues rather than integrating the issues throughout the book, implying that lesbian, gay, and bisexual people are some subgroup of people, distinct from heterosexuals in every way. The other chapters of human sexuality textbooks (ostensibly about heterosexuals) are given titles such as "Love and Relationships," "Gender Roles and Sexuality," "Communicating about Sex," and "Sexually Transmitted Diseases." None of these topics differ dramatically for lesbian, gay, or bisexual people. It would be easy to integrate all forms of sexual identity into each chapter.

If you are writing textbooks or journal articles in your specialty areas, I urge you to integrate issues of sexual identity whenever it is appropriate. Nearly every textbook concerning humans and health care should contain some reference to sexual identity, not as a problem, but as an area of human diversity that may impact health care. This may sound like an extreme suggestion, and some of you may be thinking that many human conditions have nothing to do with sexuality at all, so why should all texts discuss homosexuality? However, lesbian, gay, and bisexual people suffer from every known human disease or disorder, so when case histories or examples are provided, some could involve lesbian, gay, or bisexual clients. For example, case histories about migraine headaches could include the case of a lesbian whose migraines were precipitated or intensified by homophobic incidents at work. A case history about involving significant others in the healing process might concern a bisexual man whose male partner was trained in "healing touch." A book on death and dying could discuss the grief process in gay men whose partners have died of AIDS.

Textbooks are important, but other equally relevant components of health care education are the classroom and clinical experiences. Randall (1989) surveyed nurse educators from the Midwest and found that the majority had never discussed lesbian issues in the classroom or clinical setting, and 28% said they would be very uncomfortable teaching these issues. Ten percent thought that lesbians should not be allowed to teach in nursing schools. Wallick, Cambre, and Townsend (1992) found that the average medical school curriculum contained only about 3½ hours of discussion on homosexuality. There were regional differences with medical schools in the West having significantly more time on these issues (nearly 6 hours) compared with other regions of the country (about 2½ hours). Most of the content on homosexuality was presented within lectures on human sexuality, again perpetuating the stereotype that sexual identities are only about sex.

Often there is little education on these issues because the faculty members are uncomfortable with the issue or have had no formal training in the area. But faculty are not the only ones who can feel uncomfortable with discussions of sexual identity. Kavanagh and Kennedy (1992), writing about cultural diversity more broadly than just in terms of sexual identity, discussed the problems they encountered when they introduced topics related to diversity to their students:

> *Their lack of confidence was displayed in their communication patterns, which tended to change with topics that they considered "sensitive" areas. Overly ill-at-ease, they lowered voices, hunched shoulders, shuffled feet, diverted eyes, dropped books, got quiet, sought agreement with their ideas and feelings and sent furtive glances (often to locate members of minority groups—as if any discussion related to minority status was automatically offensive). Words they ordinarily handled with ease were stumbled over. They often became circumspect and expressed fear of "hurting feelings." Designations referring to race, ethnicity, poverty, or sexual orientation were to be avoided or reported in subdued tones. (pp. 2-3)*

Faculty will need to learn how to deal with this level of student discomfort, or their teaching may be ignored or discounted. Most faculty are unprepared to discuss issues of sexual identity, race, or gender in the classroom. These are all potentially explosive issues in our society, and educators need texts and conferences and workshops to prepare them. I use the following activity in my human development class, but it could be adapted to many other types of health care education classrooms (see Eliason & Macy, 1992). I ask students to write down the first thing that comes to their minds, whether they believe it or not, when they hear the following terms: African American, Jew, Lesbian, the Elderly, Welfare Mother, Gay Man, Bisexual, and so on. They write these words or phrases on a piece of paper and hand them in (anonymously). I tally their responses and lead a discussion of how stereotypes develop (they learned these attitudes as children generally), how powerful they are (they come to mind even though we no longer believe them), and how they might affect people who belong to the group. In my class, I talk about how being a welfare mother might affect a person's cognitive and emotional development as well as the physical growth and health of her children and herself. This exercise is nonthreatening in that the responses are anonymous and I emphasize that we cannot help what we learned as children. But it encourages the students to actively examine their own beliefs.

Clinical training opportunities should also include lesbian, gay, and bisexual issues in the form of role-playing, practice taking health histories, case discussions, rounds, and direct patient/client contact. These experiences should be structured to include sexual identity issues just as issues of race and gender are included. It is essential to prepare health care providers for the real world, which is racially and sexually diverse. We live in a sex-phobic, yet sex-obsessed culture. Many health care providers find it difficult to interview clients about any matters pertaining to sex, and homosexuality is one of the most taboo. It may help health care providers to learn to separate the public from the private. Sexual identity is the public fact—people can announce their sexual identity without revealing any information at all about their private sexual practices. To know that a person is heterosexual does not tell you anything about her/his own sexual attractions or behaviors. The public sexual identity is important for health care providers to know because it contains information about the person's potential support systems and relationships, and it suggests some specific areas of potential risk (as discussed in Chapters 7 and 8).

In many settings, the private sexual behaviors are relevant pieces of information for a health interview. Health care providers may need to have further training in human sexuality to feel comfortable interviewing clients about sexual behaviors. Think about your days as a new student—did you feel comfortable interviewing people about their bowel movements? Many things make us uncomfortable, but with practice and an understanding of their importance, we can learn to ask the questions in a matter-of-fact way that does not convey our discomfort to our clients.

These changes necessitate better education of the educators. Many current faculty members and staff development personnel need further training in issues of sexual identity so that they can:

- Learn to include lesbian, gay, and bisexual issues in their teaching in an appropriate and nonbiased manner.
- Stop perpetuating stereotypes about lesbian, gay, and bisexual people by providing misinformation or biased personal opinions.
- End the silence on issues of sexual identity and sexuality in general.

Some educators already have positive attitudes and accurate knowledge about lesbian, gay, and bisexual issues but are afraid to teach these issues to students for fear of reprisal or of being labeled as lesbian, gay, or bisexual themselves. Administrators must supply vital support by actively encouraging inclusion of these issues in the curriculum.

Policies and Procedures

Health care institutions also need to revise their policies and procedures. These include employee as well as patient/client issues. Institutional changes are slow to effect but are absolutely necessary to prevent discrimination. Again, strong administrative support is crucial in making these changes.

Employees. Health care administrators must support and guide the process of changing health care policies and procedures to reduce the potential for employee discrimination. Some questions that administrators need to ask include:

- Does the institution have a human rights statement or a nondiscrimination policy? Does that policy include sexual identity? If so, are employees who violate the policy punished?

- Are there continuing education or staff development programs for the institution/agency? If so, do they include sexual identity when appropriate? Are there specific programs about lesbian, gay, and bisexual health care needs, or fair treatment of lesbian, gay, and bisexual employees?
- Are the written materials for employees inclusive? Do some of them target lesbian, gay, and bisexual clients? Are the pictures/drawings heterosexist (only depicting heterosexual couples)? Is the language inclusive?
- Are lesbian, gay, and bisexual employees or community members represented on task forces, boards, or committees within the institution?

McNaught (1993) recommended seven strategies for eliminating discrimination of lesbian, gay, and bisexual employees. In the following discussion, these strategies are adapted to better fit the specific needs of health care institutions.

1. Formulate a written nondiscrimination policy that includes sexual identity or sexual orientation. This provides legal protection for employees and patients/clients. This type of protection is not available to most lesbian, gay, and bisexual people—only seven states (plus the District of Columbia) have sexual orientation included in their statewide human rights codes (California, Connecticut, Hawaii, Massachusetts, New Jersey, Vermont, and Wisconsin), and about 100 cities in the United States have such codes. Many large corporations have added sexual orientation to their nondiscrimination policies in recent years, and many of these companies also have domestic partner health and other benefits (e.g., AT&T, Disney World, Xerox, Microsoft, US West, and Procter & Gamble).

2. Provide a safe work environment that is free of heterosexism, racism, sexism, and other forms of bias. McNaught noted that companies usually respond in one of two ways—they are reactive or proactive. The reactive approach involves confronting prejudice when it occurs, promptly removing graffiti, or providing sensitivity training to people who have acted in a discriminatory way. The proactive approach involves providing inservice training and workshops before incidents occur, supporting lesbian, gay, and bisexual employee groups, altering the language of policies to be inclusive, promoting qualified openly gay people to positions of responsibility, and including lesbian, gay, and bisexual issues in newsletters or bulletin boards.

3. Provide institutionwide educational programs. McNaught gave three reasons for mandating or strongly encouraging participation in these programs. First, the people who most need to attend these programs will probably not come to them if participation is voluntary. Second, closeted lesbian, gay, and bisexual employees who really want to attend may be afraid to for fear of discovery. But if the program is mandated, they can safely attend. Finally, mandated programs ensure that all employees receive the same level of information. McNaught suggests conducting AIDS education programs separately from lesbian, gay, and bisexual programs, but adds that discussion of AIDS is also necessary in the programs on sexual orientation. Mandated educational programs send a strong message from the institution that discrimination will not be tolerated.

4. Provide equitable employee benefits. Because same-sex couples cannot marry in the United States, they are unfairly prevented from the tax breaks of marriage as well as the marriage benefits of employment—double discrimination. McNaught gave the following example:

> *"Larry," I said to the executive sitting in the front row, "let's pretend that you and I went to the same university, pursued the same studies, graduated with the same grades and honors, and were recruited by the same corporation. We share an office. We do the same work. We are both hailed as the best and brightest employees in the company. You get married. The next day your wife receives health care benefits from the corporation. My partner, Ray, with whom I share my life, gets nothing. Because of all the benefits your wife receives, you are getting paid more than I to do the same job. I believe that is unfair. It is not fair to me. And it is not fair to our heterosexual coworkers who for whatever reason are not married to the person with whom they share their lives." "You're right," agreed Larry. "It's not fair."* (McNaught, 1993, p. 76)

Employee benefits include health care coverage, which requires approval from the insurance carrier to add domestic partner benefits, as well as "soft" benefits that institutions control, such as bereavement and family leave, pension plans, relocation expenses, tuition grants, and access to institutional facilities such as libraries, day cares, or health clubs. Soft benefits can be added immediately, while the company negotiates with insurance carriers for "hard" benefits such as health care coverage of domestic partners.

5. Encourage lesbian, gay, and bisexual employee support groups. This backing by the institution enables employees to form support networks with their coworkers. In turn, they can provide consultation to the institution on issues that concern lesbian, gay, and bisexual clients and employees. Many large corporations have such support groups, including Lockheed, Time/Warner, and Levi Strauss. Many universities and colleges are also developing such groups. Nationwide, administrators are recognizing that empowered and supported employees are more productive. Within health care education programs, support for lesbian, gay, and bisexual students is important. Stephany (1992) noted ways that faculty members can recognize and support lesbian, gay, and bisexual nursing students. She described three sets of strategies ranging from low risk to high risk. Low-risk strategies included incorporating issues of sexual identity into the curriculum (such as discussing teen suicide risks) and showing videos about lesbian, gay, and bisexual life. Moderate-risk strategies included discussing homophobia at a faculty meeting or forming a support group for lesbian, gay, and bisexual nursing students, staff, and faculty. High-risk strategies included mandating inclusion of lesbian, gay, and bisexual issues into the curriculum, participating in gay community events, demanding domestic partner benefits in the institution and, for lesbian, gay, and bisexual faculty members, coming out to colleagues and students.

6. Ensure participation of lesbian, gay, and bisexual employees in all aspects of institutional life, from hospital unit parties to agency picnics and committees. Many institutions strive for a "family" atmosphere—if so, they should encourage all forms of family.

7. Display commitment to lesbian, gay, and bisexual employees by publicly endorsing gay rights. This can include participation in fundraisers for AIDS and gay rights organizations, having a booth or health fair at lesbian, gay, or bisexual conferences or events, donating space for meetings for gay groups, and providing time off for lesbian, gay, and bisexual employees who wish to participate in the gay health conferences or meetings. For example, Edwards (1994) reported on the efforts of Stanford University's student health center to reach out to minority students. They participated in cultural celebrations such as Black Liberation Month, Bisexual, Gay, Lesbian Awareness Days, and Cinco de Mayo. Their staff members attended events and some staff were involved on the planning committees of the events. Edwards reported that this involvement was successful in two ways. First, staff members were afforded time off from work to learn about and interact

with culturally different students and staff, furthering their education and increasing their own comfort level with diverse students. Second, their presence was affirming to the minority students on campus.

Institutions can also encourage their employees to participate in local, state, or national lesbian, gay, and bisexual professional organizations. For example, The American Association of Physicians for Human Rights (AAPHR) has more than 900 members nationwide and is committed to improving medical education and medical care for lesbian, gay, and bisexual patients/clients. The American Psychological Association has Division 44: The Society for the Psychological Study of Lesbian and Gay Issues. Many other professional organizations have lesbian, gay, and bisexual caucuses, divisions, or interest groups.

Patient Policies.   Administrators need to consider the following questions about their patient/client procedures. Many of these procedures have direct relevance to significant others:

1. Do they recognize same-sex partners as valid and legitimate?
2. Do visiting hour policies specify the relationship of the visitor; that is, do they restrict visitors to legal spouses or blood relatives? If so, they discriminate against same-sex couples.
3. Do written forms ask for marital status? If so, is there a blank for cohabitating couples? Could the item be renamed to relationship or family status and thus be made more inclusive? Lack of a cohabitation blank, or place to indicate an unmarried significant other, discriminates against same-sex couples as well as committed, but unmarried, heterosexual couples.
4. Do hospital forms have a place to indicate and store information about legal documents such as guardianship or power of attorney for health care? In the case of an emergency, do staff know they must honor these documents?
5. Do any hospital procedures require that a couple be legally married (as some artificial insemination clinics do)? What purpose does this serve, but to discriminate against unmarried couples or single people?
6. Are there policies about who can receive information about a patient or client on the phone? Do they discriminate against same-sex partners?

In the first chapter of this book, I suggested that the old equal treatment model of health care was outdated. It's time to move on. The equal treatment model considers the health care provider as a superior being, who distributes health care resources to grateful, dependent, and ignorant recipients. This condescending model needs to be replaced with a model based on health care partnership, which would also be highly individualized and culturally sensitive, and would train health care providers to seek unique solutions to individual health care problems. Instead of pushing and prodding people into narrow categories, the partnership models value uniqueness and focus on teaching critical thinking skills in health care education. A number of textbooks on culturally sensitive care are available now that provide the foundation for individualized care (see Greene, 1994; Kavanagh & Kennedy, 1992; Lassiter, 1995; Leininger, 1978, 1991; and Spector, 1991).

Health care institutions have often been resistant to change. As Kavanagh and Kennedy (1992) noted, "Members of health care disciplines have, for the most part, accepted the assumption that generalized models of care with minor adjustments for individual needs suffice, although that approach denies significant cultural and subcultural variation in health needs, expectations, and responses" (p. 32). Of course, it is impossible to teach all health care providers about every possible kind of human diversity, but it is possible to teach health care providers general skills that will allow them to adapt to each new situation. Two key skills include listening and communicating, and are discussed in the section on individual health care provider skills.

The health care institution sets the tone for the workplace. Some institutions are actively hostile to lesbian, gay, and bisexual employees and clients, most are "tolerant," some operate from benign neglect (heterosexism), and a few are truly accepting. Moving toward an accepting environment requires administrators' commitment to alter discriminatory policies and procedures and to update educational practices.

INDIVIDUAL HEALTH CARE PROVIDERS

Throughout this book I have provided concrete suggestions for individual health care providers that I will not repeat here. The following general guidelines are aimed at heterosexual health care providers who will work with lesbian, gay, and bisexual clients. Many of the same suggestions would apply to working with lesbian, gay, and bisexual coworkers. Gibson and Saunders (1994) suggested four general goals for family practice physicians who work with lesbian, gay, and bisexual clients. These four goals could easily apply to any health care discipline:

1. To improve understanding of and comfort with the realities of being a gay man or woman.
2. To have the sensitivity and skills to recognize such patients in their community and practices.
3. To project at least a nonjudgmental and preferably a supportive attitude toward these patients within the doctor-patient relationship.
4. To have adequate knowledge and skills to manage patients' unique health problems, whether personal, social, developmental, or medical. (pp. 721-722)

In previous chapters, I have described the realities of being lesbian, gay, or bisexual in contemporary U.S. cultures and have discussed potential health risks. In the remainder of this section, I will focus on concrete suggestions for health care providers committed to quality care for their clients.

I will begin with communication skills. Ask yourself, "Can I say 'lesbian, gay, or bisexual' without dropping my voice to a whisper, stuttering, or feeling uncomfortable?" If the answer is yes, that's a great start. If the answer is no, you may need practice. Role-play with a supportive coworker or family member, or practice in front of the mirror. Once you can say these words to yourself, then a supportive other, you are ready for a cross-cultural interaction. Here are a few other suggestions:

- Pay close attention to nonverbal cues such as tone of voice and facial expressions. If you feel discomfort, it will probably show in your nonverbal cues. Your lesbian, gay, or bisexual clients may seem wary or guarded—do not write them off as hostile, but consider that you may be signaling your own discomfort to them. Their reaction is a protective defense mechanism. With practice and increased knowledge about lesbian, gay, and bisexual issues, you will begin to relax and so will your clients. You can acknowledge your discomfort and admit that this kind of open communication is still new to you. Your client is likely to respect your honesty and may be more likely to be honest in return.

- Think about personal space: Do you increase the distance between yourself and the client when you discover the client's sexual identity? Do you avoid touch or feel uncomfortable when touching a lesbian, gay, or bisexual person? Think about why. Are irrational stereotypes about lesbian, gay, and bisexual people as sexual predators creeping in?

- Do you make accepting statements when a client/patient discloses sexual identity, or do you feel awkward and say nothing? The client may fear, or even expect, rejection from you. Saying nothing is akin to active rejection. Practice some accepting or acknowledging statements to avoid a shocked silence. You could ask, "Do you want me to record your sexual identity on your medical record or would you rather keep it between the two of us?" or "Do you have a significant other?" and "Does she/he have power of attorney for health care for you?"

- Avoid unprofessional voyeurism. Don't ask irrelevant questions just because you are curious. An acquaintance of mine went to a physician for an evaluation of allergies. The male physician saw a previous note on her medical chart stating that she was a lesbian and began asking her about her sexual practices. He inquired how often she and her partner used a dildo (a device that can be used for intercourse, but is only rarely used by lesbians). She replied that she had never used one, but he repeated the question three times in the course of the examination. She finally asked him what dildos had to do with her hay fever and he became somewhat hostile, but from then on he asked more relevant questions.

- Find ways that are comfortable for you to interview about sexual identity. In settings where sexual behavior is relevant, such as Ob/Gyn or STD clinics, you can ask, "Are you sexually active with men, women, both, or neither?" Then construct appropriate follow-up questions for each scenario. If sexual behavior is not relevant, you could ask about significant others, such as "Who should be included in health care decisions or information sharing?" "Is she/he an immediate family member, spouse, or life partner?" If you are comfortable, you could take a direct approach and ask, "Do you consider yourself heterosexual, lesbian, gay, or bisexual?" If you use a direct approach, don't ask this question first. Allow the client/patient to become familiar with you, and model open-mindedness and acceptance before you ask this potentially threatening question. Stephany (1993) pointed out that hospice workers need to understand their clients' sexual identity and noted that older lesbians often hide their sexuality when their caregivers visit them:

> *In hospice care this secrecy can be problematic. Is the "friend" or "roommate" listed as primary caregiver a friend or roommate (terms often used by older lesbians instead of "lover") or is she a (nonlover, never-lover) roommate or friend? Should this person be treated as a spouse or is she simply an interested party? . . . Knowing what I know now and not wishing to embarrass anyone, when I ask, I tread lightly: "You and Sharon seem very devoted to each other. Are you . . . together, a couple?" If they say yes, I ask how long they have been together. In addition to it being the next natural question to ask, it affirms their relationship and serves as an icebreaker. (p. 65)*

Can health care providers learn to be nonjudgmental? Can deep-seated prejudices be unlearned? Are some people hopelessly mired in their prejudices? The answer to all of these questions is probably yes. With accurate information, personal reflection, and positive interactions with lesbian, gay, and bisexual people, most health care providers can unlearn prejudices and learn to be nonjudgmental. But yes, some are hopelessly biased and feel too threatened to do the work required for change (for some people, challenging their stereotypes would mean challenging deeply held religious beliefs). What should be done about people who are unwilling to change their irrational and prejudicial beliefs? The ethics codes of most health care professions prohibit discriminatory care, but violations concerning sexual identity are rarely punished. Sometimes discrimination is even passively encouraged. Gaughan (1992) called homophobia "the last socially acceptable prejudice" (p. 612)—but there is no room for unscientific bias and prejudice in health care where prejudice can result in harm to clients/patients. The following sequence of events would be an effective response to a health care provider who acts out prejudice against a client/patient or coworker:

1. If the offense does not cause permanent harm to the victim (such as antigay jokes or hateful comments), the health care provider is told the behavior is unacceptable and must not be repeated.

2. If the offense is deemed more serious (refusal to provide care, threats to the victim's safety), the health care provider should be provided with educational resources, such as a workshop or counseling sessions.

3. If the behavior continues, or is of a very serious nature, the employee should be reprimanded, demoted, or fired.

Health care providers who are committed to quality care for all clients need to consider how they will deal with client confidentiality, how they will learn about their community's resources for lesbian, gay, and bisexual people, and how they can best be advocates for their lesbian, gay, and bisexual clients or patients. Since issues of sexual identity are so stigmatizing in this society, some lesbian, gay, and bisexual people have grown up without resources or information about people like them. Health care providers may actually have more information about sexual identity and health care than some lesbian, gay, and bisexual people. Don't assume that your lesbian, gay, and bisexual clients will be politically aware and knowledgeable. Do assume that you should assess their current knowledge in the same way that you assess any other client and develop a health care plan based on their individual needs.

CONCLUSION

The strategies I have described will move health care institutions and individual health care providers toward a more accepting environment for lesbian, gay, and bisexual clients, patients, and employees. These changes in the workplace can have dramatic effects on societal attitudes as well. Heterosexual clients who must answer questions about their sexual identity on health forms, who see gay-related magazines in the waiting room, or see posters of same-sex couples as well as other-sex couples on the wall, will become accustomed to these changes. As people learn that discrimination will no longer be tolerated, they will be forced to modify their behaviors, if not their attitudes. Over time, the idea that people come in different, but equally valid sexual identities will be taken for granted. The change—like the changes in racist attitudes and behaviors—will be difficult to accomplish, but it is possible and desirable in health care.

EXERCISE: A GLIMPSE OF LESBIAN, GAY, OR BISEXUAL LIFE

This activity was suggested by McNaught (1993) in his book on gay issues in the workplace. If you are a heterosexual, go to a bookstore in your neighborhood and ask the clerk for a book about lesbian, gay, and bisexual issues. Note how it feels (did your voice shake? Did you lower your voice so other customers could not hear you?). Were you afraid the clerk or customers would think you were lesbian, gay, or bisexual? How did the clerk react to you? Look for verbal and nonverbal clues.

Now take that book (or this one), to a public place such as a coffee shop or the employee lounge where you work. Read the book when others are present. Did you feel a strong urge to cover the title? Did any coworkers or strangers look at you in curiosity? If you were actually able to do this exercise, you will have some small appreciation for what it feels like to be lesbian, gay, or bisexual in our culture. If you were unable to do this exercise because it felt too threatening or uncomfortable, you will have some sense of why so many lesbian, gay, and bisexual people stay in the closet.

CHAPTER TEN

Afterword

I HOPE THAT I HAVE sparked your interest in lesbian, gay, and bisexual health care issues, or incurred your rage at the injustices in health care, or emboldened you to speak out against homophobic remarks at work. I hope I have challenged the stereotypes about lesbian, gay, or bisexual people, and heightened your awareness of their difficulties in negotiating the treacherous health care system. I hope that lesbian, gay, and bisexual readers feel more informed about their health care needs, and become committed to advocating for their own health care rights.

If nothing else, this book exposes the serious gaps in our knowledge. There is a clear need for education of students and faculty alike, for changes in health care policy, and for further research. This review of the health care literature strongly suggests that the following areas are among the many that need study:

- Identify successful interventions for different kinds of negative attitudes: How can people change irrational beliefs? ignorance? feelings of hatred?
- Define the link between attitudes and behaviors: How do negative attitudes manifest in health care provider behaviors?
- Study the ways that homophobia affects health: Does health care provider discomfort affect patient compliance? Does it affect the patient's ability to understand and retain health care teaching?
- Examine the best ways to teach students issues of sexuality: Should it be in separate courses or integrated throughout the curriculum? How much education is needed?

- Address the negative attitudes of practicing health care providers: How can they be reached? Continuing education programs? Inservice education? Unit discussion groups? Should programs be mandated or voluntary?

- Discover ways that health care providers can reduce the risks for suicide in lesbian, gay, and bisexual teens and young adults.

- Study more carefully the disclosure process: How can we create accepting and inclusive environments that allow for disclosure?

- Examine the consequences of internalized homophobia and determine its role in physical and mental health of lesbian, gay, and bisexual people, then develop interventions to reduce or eliminate it.

- Discuss the feasibility of expanding the AIDS risk categories of the CDC to reflect the realities of sexual behavior.

- Begin to discuss the issues of transgendered people along with discussions of sexuality. People who are transgendered (deviate from societal norms for the behavior, appearance, or mannerisms assigned to their biological sex) face many of the same forms of harassment and discrimination in health care as do lesbian, gay, and bisexual people. Additionally, many transgendered people are also lesbian, gay, or bisexual in their sexual identities. Transgender health care rights need to be considered. The first step would involve removing gender identity disorder from the DSM-IV.

- Study lesbian, gay, and bisexual families more closely: How can we teach parents to interact with schools, pediatricians, and other institutions their children will attend, and how do we help children cope with potential teasing or questions from their peers and teachers?

- Devote more resources to the study of breast cancer in all women, but particularly to better definition of the risk factors and education of lesbians about breast health. Breast cancer must be considered as an epidemic; a crisis in health care.

These are only a few of the studies that are needed. Until much more research is done, health care providers must rely on the scant data that we already have, or base recommendations on findings from presumably heterosexual samples, which may or may not apply.

In addition to more and better designed research, lesbian, gay, and bisexual people need to come forward and talk about health care experiences. Lesbian, gay, and bisexual health care providers need to provide positive role models for clients, patients, coworkers, and students in their professions. Some people still don't believe that there are lesbian, gay, and bisexual physicians, nurses, dentists, social workers, speech therapists, physical therapists, dietiticians, and physician assistants. These professionals need to become visible.

When lesbian, gay, and bisexual patients have bad experiences, they need to complain and demand equitable health care. Many health care providers don't even know when they have offended or hurt or silenced a client or patient, because the person's sexual identity is invisible. Unless the injured person tells them, they will continue to make the same heterosexist and homophobic mistakes. Another reason for speaking out is to share health care experiences with other lesbian, gay, and bisexual people. We sometimes feel isolated and alone when facing the health care system, because we don't have a road map for negotiating that system. When we suffer discrimination without complaint, we not only hurt ourselves, but harm other lesbian, gay, and bisexual clients and patients as well. Audre Lorde, an African American lesbian poet and activist died of breast cancer in 1992. Soon after her diagnosis and mastectomy in 1977, she wrote:

> *I have come to believe over and over again that what is most important to me must be spoken, made verbal and shared, even at the risk of having it bruised or misunderstood. That the speaking profits me, beyond any other effect. I am standing here as a black lesbian poet, and the meaning of all that waits upon the fact that I am still alive, and might not have been. Less than two months ago, I was told by two doctors, one female and one male, that I would have to have breast surgery, and that there was a 60 to 80 percent chance that the tumor was malignant. . . . In becoming forcibly and essentially aware of my mortality, and of what I wished and wanted for my life, however short it might be, priorities and omissions became strongly etched in a merciless light and what I most regretted were my silences. Of what had I ever been afraid? . . . My silences had not protected me. Your silence will not protect you. . . . What are the words you do not yet have? What do you need to say? What are the tyrannies you swallow day by day and attempt to make*

your own, until you will sicken and die of them, still in silence.
Perhaps for some of you here today, I am the face of one of your
fears. Because I am woman, because I am black, because I am
lesbian, because I am myself, a black woman warrior poet
doing my work, come to ask you, are you doing yours? (Audre
Lorde, 1980, pp. 19-21)

If there is one message that I want you to take away from this book,
it is to break the silences. Talk about lesbian, gay, and bisexual issues in
the workplace and in the classroom. Encourage your lesbian, gay, and
bisexual patients, clients, and coworkers to be open about their lives.
Talk about the things that are difficult for us all—the breast cancer epidemic in women, the AIDS epidemic that will soon affect each one of
us personally if it doesn't already, the loss of our lesbian, gay, or bisexual friend or family member to suicide or hate crimes, and the pain
when our families or relationships are not validated. Only by breaking
the silence can the healing process begin.

Sample Durable Power of Attorney for Health Care*

I, _____ , hereby appoint:

Name _____

Home address _____

_____

Home telephone number _____

Work telephone number _____

as my agent to make health care decisions for me if and when I am unable to make my own health care decisions. This gives my agent the power to consent to giving, withholding, or stopping my health care, treatment, service, or diagnostic procedure. My agent also has the authority to talk with health care personnel, get information, and sign forms necessary to carry out those decisions.

If the person named as my agent is not available or is unable to act as my agent, then I appoint the following person(s) to serve in the order listed below:

(list name, address, and phone numbers of 1 or more other people)

By this document I intend to create a power of attorney for health care which shall take effect upon my incapacity to make my own health care decisions and shall continue during that incapacity.

My agent shall make health care decisions as I direct below or as I make known to her or him in some other way.

*This is a generic form: Please consult a reliable source of information for the specific requirements of the state in which you live.

Statement of Desires concerning life-prolonging care, treatment, services, and procedures:

_____

_____

_____

_____

_____

Special provisions and limitations:

_____

_____

_____

_____

_____

By signing here I indicate that I understand the purpose and effect of this document.

Date _____

Current home address_____

_____

_____

Signature

Witnesses:

I declare that the person who signed or acknowledged this document is personally known to me, that she/he signed or acknowledged this durable power of attorney in my presence, and that she/he appears to be of sound mind and under no duress, fraud, or undue influence. I am not the person appointed as agent by this document, nor am I the patient's health care provider, nor an employee of the patient's health care provider.

First Witness

Signature _____

Home address _____

_____

Print name _____

Date _____

Second Witness

Signature _____

Home address _____

_____

Print name _____

Date _____

(At least one of the above witnesses must also sign the following declaration.)

I further declare that I am not related to the patient by blood, marriage, or adoption, and, to the best of my knowledge, I am not entitled to any part of her/his estate under a will now existing or by operation of law.

Signature _____

Print name _____

References

Aarons, L. (1995). *Prayers for Bobby: A mother's coming to terms with the suicide of her gay son.* New York: HarperCollins.

Achtenberg, R. (1988). Preserving and protecting the families of lesbians and gay men. In M. Shernoff & W. A. Scott (Eds.), *The sourcebook on lesbian/gay health care* (pp. 237-245). Washington, DC: National Lesbian and Gay Health Foundation.

Adelman, M. (1990). Stigma, gay lifestyles, and adjustment to aging: A study of later-life gay men and lesbians. *Journal of Homosexuality, 20*(3/4), 7-32.

Alexander, R., & Fitzpatrick, J. (1990). Variables influencing nurses' attitudes toward AIDS and AIDS patients. *AIDS Patient Care, 4,* 315-320.

Alpert, H. (1988). *We are everywhere: Writings by and about lesbian parents.* Freedom, CA: Crossing Press.

Alyson, S. (Ed.). (1991). *Young, gay, and proud* (3rd ed.). Boston: Alyson.

American Psychiatric Association. (1994). *Diagnostic and statistical manual of mental disorders* (4th ed.). Washington, DC: Author.

Angel, C. (1993). AIDS and the African American PWA. In B. Hunter (Ed.), *Sojourner: Black gay voices in the age of AIDS.* New York: Other Country.

Anzaldua, G. (1987). Borderlands/La Frontera: The new mestiza. San Francisco, CA: Spinsters/Aunt Lute.

Aura, J. (1985). *Women's social support: A comparison of lesbians and heterosexuals.* Unpublished doctoral dissertation, University of California, Los Angeles.

Badgett, L. (1996). Choices and chances: Is coming out at work a rational choice? In B. Beemyn & M. Eliason (Eds.), *Queer studies: A lesbian, gay, bisexual, and transgender anthology.* New York: New York University Press.

Bailey, J. M., Miller, J., & Willerman, L. (1993). Maternally rated childhood gender: Nonconformity in homosexuals and heterosexuals. *Archives of Sexual Behavior, 22*(5), 461-469.

Bailey, J. M., & Pillard, R. C. (1991). A genetic study of male sexual orientation. *Archives of General Psychiatry, 48,* 1089-1096.

Barrett, R. L., & Robinson, B. E. (1990). *Gay fathers.* Lexington, MA: Lexington Books.

Bart, P. (1994). Introduction. In J. Penelope (Ed.), *Out of the class closet: Lesbians speak.* Freedom, CA: Crossing Press.

Beam, J. (1986). *In the life: A black gay anthology.* Boston: Alyson.

Beck, E. T., (Ed.). (1982). *Nice Jewish girls: A Jewish lesbian anthology.* Watertown, MA: Persephone Press.

Behney, R. (1995). Research: Gauging the aging network's response. *Aging Today,* September/October, 8.

Belcastro, P. A. (1982). A comparison of latent sexual behavior patterns between raped and never raped females. *Victimology, 7*(1-4), 224-230.

Bell, A. P., & Weinberg, M. S. (1978). *Homosexualities: A study of diversity among men and women.* New York: Simon & Schuster.

Benkov, L. (1994). *Reinventing the family: Lesbian and gay parents.* New York: Crown.

Berger, R. (1980). Psychological adaptation of the older homosexual male. *Journal of Homosexuality, 5,* 161-175.

Bergler, E. (1956). *Homosexuality: Disease or way of Life?* New York: Hill and Wang.

Berrill, K. (1992). Anti-gay violence and victimization in the United States: An overview. In G. Herek & K. Berrill (Eds.), *Hate crimes.* Newbury Park, CA: Sage.

Bevier, P. J., Chiasson, M. A., Hefferman, R. T., & Catro, K. G. (1995). Women at sexually transmitted disease clinics who reported same-sex contact: Their HIV seroprevalence and risk behaviors. *American Journal of Public Health, 85,* 1366-1371.

Bidwell, R. J. (1988). The gay and lesbian teen: A case of denied adolescence. *Journal of Pediatric Health Care, 2*(1), 3-8.

Bierley, M. (1985). Prejudice toward contemporary outgroups as a generalized attitude. *Journal of Applied Social Psychology, 15,* 189-199.

Bigner, J. J., & Jacobsen, R. B. (1989a). Parenting behaviors of homosexual and heterosexual fathers. *Journal of Homosexuality, 18,* 173-182.

Bigner, J. J., & Jacobsen, R. B. (1989b). The value of children to gay and heterosexual fathers. *Journal of Homosexuality, 18,* 163-172.

Bloomfield, K. (1993). A comparison of alcohol consumption between lesbians and heterosexual women in an urban population. *Drug and Alcohol Dependence, 33,* 257-269.

Blumenfeld, W. (1992). *Homophobia: How we all pay the price.* Boston: Alyson.

Blumenfeld, W. (1996). History/hysteria: Parallel representations of Jews and gays, lesbians, and bisexuals. In B. Beemyn & M. Eliason (Eds.), *Queer studies: A lesbian, gay, bisexual, & transgender anthology.* New York: New York University Press.

Blumenfeld, W., & Raymond, D. (1988). *Looking at gay and lesbian life.* Boston: Beacon Press.

Blumenfield, M., Smith, P., Milazzo, J., Seropian, S., & Wormser, G. P. (1987). Survey of nurses working with AIDS patients. *General Hospital Psychiatry, 9,* 58-63.

Blumstein, P., & Schwartz, P. (1983). *American couples: Money, work, sex.* New York: Morrow.

Borhek, M. (1983). *Coming out to parents: A two way survival guide for lesbians and gay men and their parents.* New York: Pilgrim Press.

Boswell, J. (1980). *Christianity, social tolerance and homosexuality.* Chicago: University of Chicago Press.

Boswell, J. (1994). *Same-sex unions in premodern Europe.* New York: Villard.

Bozett, F. W. (1982). Heterogeneous couples in heterosexual marriages: Gay men and straight women. *Journal of Marital and Sexual Therapy, 8,* 81-89.

Bozett, F. W. (1987). Children of gay fathers. In F. W. Bozett (Ed.), *Gay and lesbian parents* (pp. 39-57). New York: Praeger.

Bozett, F. W. (1988). Social control of identity by children of gay fathers. *Western Journal of Nursing Research, 10,* 550-565.

Bradford, J., & Ryan, C. (1988). *National Lesbian Health Care Survey: Final report.* Washington, DC: National Lesbian and Gay Foundation.

Bradford, J., & Ryan, C. (1991). Who we are: Health concerns of middle-aged lesbians. In B. Sang, J. Warshow, & A. Smith (Eds.), *Lesbians at midlife: The creative transition.* San Francisco: Spinsters.

Bradford, J., Ryan, C., & Rothblum, E. D. (1994). National Lesbian Health Care Survey: Implications for mental health care. *Journal of Consulting and Clinical Psychology, 62*(2), 228-242.

Brannock, J. C., & Chapman, B. E. (1990). Negative sexual experiences with men among heterosexual women and lesbians. *Journal of Homosexuality, 19*(1), 105-110.

Brenner, C. (1992). Survivors story: Eight bullets. In G. Herek & K. Berrill (Eds.), *Hate crimes.* Newbury Park, CA: Sage.

Brossart, G. (1979). The gay patient: What you should be doing. *RN, 42*(4), 50-52.

Brownfain, J. J. (1985). A study of the married bisexual male: Paradox and resolution. *Journal of Homosexuality, 11*(1/2), 173-188.

Brownsworth, V. (1995). ER: Queer style. *Deneuve: The Lesbian Magazine, 5*(5), 50.

Bryant, A. S., & Demian, R. (1994). Relationship characteristics of American gay and lesbian couples: Findings from a national survey. *Journal of Gay and Lesbian Social Services, 1,* 101-117.

Buenting, J. (1992). Health life-styles of lesbians and heterosexual women. *Health Care for Women International, 13*(2), 75-82.

Buhrich, N., & Loke, C. (1988). Homosexuality, suicide and parasuicide in Australia. *Journal of Homosexuality, 15*(1/2), 113-129.

Burke, P. (1993). *Family values: Two moms and their son.* New York: Random House.

Cameron, P. (1988). Kinsey sex surveys. *Science, 240,* 867.

Cameron, P., Proctor, K., Coburn, W., Jr., & Forde, N. (1985). Sexual orientation and sexually transmitted disease. *Nebraska Medical Journal, 70,* 292-299.

Carballo-Diéguez, A. (1995). The sexual identity and behavior of Puerto Rican men who have sex with men. In G. Herek & B. Greene (Eds.), *AIDS, identity, and community: The HIV epidemic and lesbians and gay men.* Thousand Oaks, CA: Sage.

Card, C. (1990). Why homophobia? *Hypatia, 5,* 110-117.

Carlson, H. M., & Baxter, L. A. (1984). Androgyny, depression, and self-esteem in Irish homosexual and heterosexual males and females. *Sex roles, 10,* 457-467.

Carlson, H. M., & Steuer, J. (1985). Age, sex-role categorization and psychological health in American homosexual and heterosexual men and women. *Journal of Social Work, 125,* 203-211.

Cass, V. C. (1979). Homosexual identity formation: A theoretical model. *Journal of Homosexuality, 4,* 219-236.

Cass, V. C. (1984a). Homosexual identity: A concept in need of definition. *Journal of Homosexuality, 9,* 105-126.

Cass, V. C. (1984b). Homosexual identity formation: Testing a theoretical model. *Journal of Sex Research, 20,* 143-167.

Chaimowitz, G. A. (1991). Homophobia among psychiatric residents, family practice residents and psychiatric faculty. *Canadian Journal of Psychiatry, 36*(3), 206-209.

Chan, C. S. (1989). Issues of identity development among Asian-American lesbians and gay men. *Journal of Counseling and Development, 68,* 16-20.

Chapman, B., & Brannock, J. (1987). Proposed model of lesbian identity development: An empirical examination. *Journal of Homosexuality, 14*(3/4), 69-80.

Charbonneau, C., & Lander, P. (1991). Redefining sexuality: Women becoming lesbian in midlife. In B. Sang, J. Warshow, & A. Smith (Eds.), *Lesbians at midlife.* San Francisco, CA: Spinsters.

Christie, D., & Young, M. (1986). Self-concept of lesbian and heterosexual women. *Psychological Reports, 59,* 1279-1282.

Chu, S., Buehler, J., Fleming, P., & Berkelman, R. (1990). Epidemiology of reported cases of AIDS in lesbians, United States 1980-89. *American Journal of Public Health, 80*(11), 1380-1381.

Clark, T. R. (1975). Homosexuality and psychopathology in nonpatient males. *American Journal of Psychoanalysis, 35,* 163-168.

Clunis, D. M., & Green, G. D. (1993). *Lesbian couples.* Seattle, WA: Seal Press.

Cochran, S., & Mays, V. (1988). Disclosure of sexual preference to physicians by black lesbian and bisexual women. *Western Journal of Medicine, 149,* 616-619.

Cochran, S., & Mays, V. (1994). Depressive distress among homosexually active African American men and women. *American Journal of Psychiatry, 151*(4), 524-529.

Cohen, T. (1983). The incestuous family revisited. *Social Casework, 64*(3), 154-161.

Cole, E., & Rothblum, E. (1991). Lesbian sex at midlife: As good or better than ever. In B. Sang, J. Warshow, & A. Smith (Eds.), *Lesbians at midlife.* San Francisco, CA: Spinsters.

Cole, F. L., & Slocumb, E. M. (1993). Nurses' attitudes towards patients with AIDS. *Journal of Advanced Nursing, 18,* 1112-1117.

Cole, F. L., & Slocumb, E. M. (1994). Mode of acquiring AIDS and nurses' intention to provide care. *Research in Nursing and Health, 17,* 303-309.

Cole, R., & Cooper, S. (1990, December/1991, January). Lesbian exclusion from HIV/AIDS education. *SIECUS Report, 19*(2), 18-23.

Coleman, E. (1985a). Bisexual women in marriages. *Journal of Homosexuality, 11*(1/2), 87-99.

Coleman, E. (1985b). Integration of male bisexuality and marriage. *Journal of Homosexuality, 11*(1/2), 189-207.

Coleman, E., & Remafedi, G. (1989). Gay, lesbian, and bisexual adolescents: A critical challenge to counselors. *Journal of Counseling and Development, 68,* 36-40.

Committee on Adolescence. (1993). Homosexuality and adolescence. *Pediatrics, 92*(4), 631-634.

Comstock, G. (1991). *Violence against lesbians and gay men.* New York: Columbia University Press.

Conerly, G. (1996). The politics of black lesbian and gay identity. In B. Beemyn & M. J. Eliason (Eds.), *Queer studies: A lesbian, gay, bisexual and transgender anthology.* New York: New York University Press.

Connell, R., Crawford, J., Dowsett, G., Kippax, S., Sinnott, V., Rodden, P., Berg, R., Baxter, D., & Watson, L. (1990). Danger and context: Unsafe anal sexual practice among homosexual and bisexual men. *Australian and New Zealand Journal of Sociology, 26,* 187-208.

Cotton, P. (1992). Attacks on homosexual persons may be increasing, but many bashings still aren't reported to police. *Journal of the American Medical Association, 267*(22), 2999-3000.

Countryman, L. W. (1988). *Dirt, greed, and sex: Sexual ethics in the New Testament and their implications for today.* Philadelphia: Fortress Press.

Cramer, D. W., & Roach, A. S. (1988). Coming out to mom and dad: A study of gay males and their relationships with their parents. *Journal of Homosexuality, 15*(3/4), 79-91.

Curry, H., & Clifford, D. (1991). *A legal guide for lesbian and gay couples* (6th ed.). Berkeley, CA: Nolo Press.

Curtin, L. L. (1994). Lesbian, single and geriatric women: To breed or not to breed? *Nursing Management, 25*(3), 14-16.

Dardick, L., & Grady, K. (1980). Openness between gay persons and health professionals. *Annals of Internal Medicine, 93*(Part I), 115-119.

D'Augelli, A. R., & Hershberger, S. L. (1993). Lesbian, gay and bisexual youth in community settings: Personal challenges and mental health problems. *American Journal of Community Psychology, 21*(4), 421-448.

Dawson, J. M., Fitzpatrick, R. M., Reeves, G., Boulton, M., McLean, J., Hart, G., & Brookes, M. (1994). Awareness of sexual partners' HIV status as an influence upon high-risk sexual behavior among gay men. *AIDS, 8*(6), 837–841.

Dean, L. (1995). Psychosocial stressors in a panel of New York City gay men during the AIDS epidemic, 1985–1991. In G. Herek & B. Greene (Eds.), *AIDS, identity, and community: The HIV epidemic and lesbians and gay men.* Thousand Oaks, CA: Sage.

DeCecco, J., & Parker, D. (1995). The biology of homosexuality: Sexual orientation or sexual preference. *Journal of Homosexuality, 28*(1/2), 1–28.

Deevy, S. (1990). Older lesbian women: An invisible minority. *Journal of Gerontological Nursing, 16*(5), 35–37.

Deevy, S. (1993). Lesbian self-disclosure: Strategies for success. *Journal of Psychosocial Nursing, 31*(4), 21–26.

Degen, K., & Waitkevicz, H. (1982). Lesbian health issues. *British Journal Sex and Medicine,* May, 40–47.

D'Emilio, J., & Freedman, E. (1988). *Intimate matters: A history of sexuality in America.* New York: Harper and Row.

Denenberg, R. (1992). Invisible women: Lesbians and health care. *Health Policy Advisory Center Bulletin, 22*(1), 14–21.

Diamond, M. (1993). Homosexuality and bisexuality in different populations. *Archives of Sexual Behavior, 22*(4), 291–310.

Douglas, C. J., Kalman, C. M., & Kalman, T. P. (1985). Homophobia among physicians and nurses: An empirical study. *Hospital and Community Psychiatry, 36*(12), 1309–1311.

Duberman, M. (1993). *Stonewall.* New York, NY: Dutton.

Due, L. (1995). *Joining the tribe: Growing up gay and lesbian in the 90s.* New York: Anchor Books.

Duffy, S. M., & Rusbult, C. E. (1985/1986). Satisfaction and commitment in homosexual and heterosexual relationships. *Journal of Homosexuality, 12*(2), 1–23.

Duggan, L. (1992). Scholars and sense. *Village Voice Literary Supplement,* June, 27.

Dunn, F. (1993). When to fight, when to care. In B. Hunter (Ed.), *Sojourner: Black gay voices in the age of AIDS.* New York: Other Country.

Dworkin, S., & Guitierrez, F. (1989). Counselors be aware clients come in every size, shape, color, and sexual orientation. *Journal of Counseling and Development, 68,* 6–10.

Editors, Harvard Law Review. (1990). *Sexual orientation and the law.* Cambridge, MA: Harvard University Press.

Edwards, S. (1994, March). The student health center as multicultural catalyst. *Journal of College Health, 42,* 225–228.

Ekstrand, M., & Coates, T. (1990). Maintenance of safer sexual behaviors and predictors of risky sex: The San Francisco Men's Health Study. *American Journal of Public Health, 80,* 973–977.

Eliason, M. J. (1993a). AIDS-related stigma and homophobia: Implications for nursing education. *Nurse Educator, 18*(6), 27–30.

Eliason, M. J. (1993b). Cultural diversity in nursing care: The lesbian, gay, or bisexual client. *Journal of Transcultural Nursing, 5*(1), 14-20.

Eliason, M. J. (1995). Attitudes about lesbians and gay men: A review and implications for social service training. *Journal of Gay and Lesbian Social Services, 2,* 73-90.

Eliason, M. J. (1996a). *Heterosexual undergraduate students' attitudes about bisexuality.* Iowa City, IA: University of Iowa College of Nursing.

Eliason, M. J. (1996b). An inclusive model of lesbian identity. *Journal of Lesbian, Gay, and Bisexual Identity, 1*(1), 3-9.

Eliason, M. J. (1996c). The campus climate for lesbian, gay, and bisexual university members. *Journal of Psychology and Human Sexuality, 000,* 000-000.

Eliason, M. J. (1996d). Identity formation for lesbian, bisexual and gay persons: Beyond a minority view. *Journal of Homosexuality, 30*(2), 35-62.

Eliason, M. J., Donelan, C., & Randall, C. (1992). Lesbian stereotypes. *Health Care for Women International, 13,* 131-144.

Eliason, M. J., & Macy, N. (1992). A classroom activity to introduce cultural diversity. *Nurse Educator, 17,* 32-36.

Eliason, M. J., & Morgan, K. (1996a). *How lesbians define themselves.* Iowa City, IA: University of Iowa College of Nursing.

Eliason, M. J., & Morgan, K. (1996b). Therapy usage and political activity in lesbians. *Women and Therapy, 000,* 000-000.

Eliason, M. J., & Morgan, K. (1996c). *Lesbians and physical health care seeking.* Iowa City, IA: University of Iowa College of Nursing.

Eliason, M., & Raheim, S. (1996). Categorical measurement of attitudes toward lesbian, gay and bisexual people. *Journal of Gay and Lesbian Social Services, 000,* 000-000.

Eliason, M., & Randall, C. (1991). Lesbian phobia in nursing students. *Western Journal of Nursing Research, 13,* 383-374.

Ernulf, K., & Innala, S. (1987). The relationship between affective and cognitive components of homophobic reaction. *Archives of Sexual Behavior, 16,* 501-509.

Espín, O. M. (1987). Issues of identity in the psychology of lesbian latinas. In Boston Lesbian Psychologies Collective (Eds.), *Lesbian psychologies: Explorations and Challenges* (pp. 35-51). Urbana: University of Illinois Press.

Faderman, L. (1984). The "new gay" lesbian. *Journal of Homosexuality, 10*(3/4), 85-95.

Fairchild, B., & Hayward, N. (1989). *Now that you know: What every parent should know about homosexuality.* New York: Harcourt, Brace & Jovanovich.

Falk, P. (1989). Lesbian mothers: Psychosexual assumptions in family law. *American Psychologist, 44,* 941-947.

Feierman, J. (1990). *Pedophilia: Biosocial dimensions.* New York: Springer-Verlag.

Fertitta, S. (1987). *Never married women in the middle years: A comparison of lesbians and heterosexuals.* Paper presented at the Annual Conference of the American Psychological Association, New York.

Festinger, L. (1964). Behavioral support for opinion change. *Public Opinion Quarterly, 28,* 404-417.

Ficarrotto, T. (1990). Racism, sexism and erotophobia: Attitudes of heterosexuals toward homosexuals. *Journal of Homosexuality, 19,* 111-116.

Fifield, L. H. (1975). *On my way to nowhere: Alienated, isolated, drunk: An analysis of gay alcohol abuse and an evaluation of alcoholism rehabilitation services for the Los Angeles gay community.* Los Angeles, CA: Gay Community Services Center.

Finnegan, D. G., & McNally, E. B. (1987). *Dual identities: Counseling chemically dependent gay men and lesbians.* Center City, MN: Hazelden.

Fish, T. A., & Rye, B. (1991). Attitudes toward a homosexual or heterosexual person with AIDS. *Journal of Applied Social Psychology, 21*(8), 651-667.

Fletcher, J. L. (1984). Homosexuality: Kick and kickback. *Southern Medical Journal, 77*(2), 149-150.

Forstein, M. (1988). Homophobia: An overview. *Psychiatric Annals, 18,* 33-36.

Foucault, M. (1969). *The History of Sexuality* (Vol. 1). New York: Random House.

Friend, R. A. (1987). The individual and social psychology of aging: Clinical implications for lesbians and gay men. *Journal of Homosexuality, 14,* 307-331.

Garber, M. (1995). *Vice versa: Bisexuality and the eroticism of every day life.* New York: Simon & Schuster.

Garnets, L. D., Herek, G. M., & Levy, B. (1990). Violence and victimization of lesbians and gay men: Mental health consequences. *Journal of Interpersonal Violence, 5,* 366-383.

Garnets, L. D., & Kimmel, D. C. (1993). Lesbian and gay male dimensions in the psychological study of human diversity. In L. D. Garnets & D. C. Kimmel (Eds.), *Psychological perspectives on lesbian and gay male experiences* (pp. 1-51). New York: Columbia University Press.

Gaughan, T. (1992). The last socially acceptable prejudice. *American Libraries, 612.*

Gebhard, P. H. (1972). Incidence of overt homosexuality in the U.S. and Western Europe. In J. J. Livengood (Ed.), *NIMH Task Force on Homosexuality: Final Report and Background Papers* (DHEW Public. No. HSM 72-9116). Rockville, MD: National Institute of Mental Health.

Geddes, V. (1994). Lesbian expectations and experiences with family doctors. *Canadian Family Physician, 40,* 908-920.

Gibson, G., & Saunders, D. (1994). Gay patients. *Canadian Family Physician, 40,* 721-725.

Gibson, P. (1994). Gay male and lesbian youth suicide. In G. Remafedi (Ed.), *Death by Denial: Studies of suicide in gay and lesbian teenagers.* Boston, MA: Alyson.

Gillow, K. E., & Davis, L. L. (1987). Lesbian stress and coping methods. *Journal of Psychosocial Nursing, 25*(9), 28-32.

Glaus, K. O. (1989). Alcoholism, chemical dependency and the lesbian client. *Women and Therapy, 8,* 131-144.

Glenn, C. (1991). In my own space. In E. Hemphill (Ed.), *Brother to brother: New writings by black gay men.* Boston: Alyson.

Gochros, J. S. (1989). *When husbands come out of the closet.* New York: Haworth Press.

Goff, J. L. (1990). Sexual confusion among certain college males. *Adolescence, 25,* 599-614.

Golombok, S., Spencer, A., & Rutter, M. (1983). Children in lesbian and single-parent households: Psychosexual and psychiatric appraisal. *Journal of Child Psychology and Psychiatry, 24*(4), 551-572.

Gonsiorek, J. C. (1991). The empirical basis for the demise of the illness model of homosexuality. In J. Gonsiorek & J. Weinrich (Eds.), *Homosexuality: Research implications for public policy* (pp. 115-136). Newbury Park, CA: Sage.

Gonsiorek, J. C., & Weinrich, J. D. (1991). The definition and scope of sexual orientation. In J. C. Gonsiorek & J. D. Weinrich (Eds.), *Homosexuality: Research implications for public policy* (pp. 1-12). Newbury Park, CA: Sage.

Gottman, J. S. (1990). Children of gay and lesbian parents. In F. W. Bozett & M. B. Sussman (Eds.), *Homosexuality and family relations* (pp. 177-196). New York: Harrington Park Press.

Gramick, J. (1984). Developing a lesbian identity. In T. Darty & S. Potter (Eds.), *Women-identified women* (pp. 31-44). Palo Alto, CA: Mayfield.

Green, R. (1978). Sexual identity of 37 children raised by homosexual or transsexual parents. *American Journal of Psychiatry, 135,* 692-697.

Green, R. (1985). Gender identity in childhood and later sexual orientation: Follow-up of 78 males. *American Journal of Psychiatry, 142,*(3), 339-341.

Green, R. (1987). *The "sissy boy syndrome" and the development of homosexuality.* New Haven, CT: Yale University Press.

Green, R., Mandel, J. B., Hotvedt, M. E., Gray, J., & Smith, L. (1986). Lesbian mothers and their children: A comparison with solo parent heterosexual mothers and their children. *Archives of Sexual Behavior, 15*(2), 167-185.

Greene, B. (1986). When the therapist is white and the patient is black: Considerations for psychotherapy in the feminist heterosexual and lesbian communities. In D. Howard (Ed.), *The Dynamics of feminist therapy* (pp. 41-65). New York: Haworth Press.

Greene, B. (1994). Ethnic-minority lesbians and gay men: Mental health and treatment issues. *Journal of Consulting and Clinical Psychology, 62*(2), 243-251.

Grellert, E. A., Newcomb, M. D., & Bentler, P. M. (1982). Childhood play activities of male and female homosexuals and heterosexuals. *Archives of Sexual Behavior, 11*(6), 451-478.

Griffin, C., Wirth, M., & Wirth, A. (1986). *Beyond acceptance: Parents of lesbians and gay talk about their experience.* Englewood Cliffs, NJ: Prentice-Hall.

Gundlach, R. H., & Reiss, B. F. (1967). Birth order and sex of siblings in sample of lesbians and nonlesbians. *Psychological Reports, 20*(1), 61-62.

Haaga, D. (1991). "Homophobia?" *Journal of Social Behavior and Personality, 6,* 171-174.

Haldeman, D. C. (1994). The practice and ethics of sexual orientation conversion therapy. *Journal of Consulting and Clinical Psychology, 62*(2), 221-227.

Hall, J. (1994). Lesbians recovering from alcohol problems: An ethnographic study of health care experiences. *Nursing Research, 43*(4), 238-244.

Hall, M. (1978). Lesbian families: Cultural and clinical issues. *Social Work, 23,* 380-385.

Hall, M. (1989). Private expression in the public domain: Lesbians in organizations. In J. Mearn, D. L. Sheppard, P. Tancred-Sheriff, & G. Burrell (Eds.), *The sexuality of organization* (pp. 125-138). Newbury Park, CA: Sage.

Hamer, D. H., & Copeland, P. (1994). *The science of desire: The search for the gay gene and the biology of behavior.* New York: Simon & Schuster.

Hamer, D. H., Hu, S., Magnuson, V. L., Hu, N., & Pattatucci, A. M. (1993). A linkage between DNA markers on the X chromosome and male sexual orientation. *Science, 261,* 321-327.

Haring, J. H., & Lind, L. J. (1992). Attitudes of dental hygiene students toward individuals with AIDS. *Journal of Dental Education, 56*(2), 128-130.

Harris, M. B., Nightengale, J., & Owen, N. (1995). Health care professionals' experience, knowledge, and attitudes concerning homosexuality. *Journal of Gay and Lesbian Social Services, 2,* 91-107.

Harrison, M., Fusilier, M. R., & Worley, J. K. (1994). Development of a measure of nurses' aides attitudes and conservative views. *Psychological Reports, 74,* 1043-1048.

Harry, J. (1982). *Gay children grown up.* New York: Praeger.

Harry, J. (1983). Defeminization and adult psychological well-being among male homosexuals. *Archives of Sexual Behavior, 12,* 1-19.

Harvey, S. M., Carr, C., & Bernheine, S. (1989). Lesbian mothers: Health care experiences. *Journal of Nurse-Midwifery, 34*(3), 115-199.

Hassel, W. (1992). Survivors story. In G. Herek & K. Berrill (Eds.), *Hate crimes.* Thousand Oaks, CA: Sage.

Hatfield, L. (1989, June 5). Method of polling. *San Francisco Examiner, A20.*

Hayes, R., Kegeles, S., & Coates, T. (1990). High HIV risk-taking among young gay men. *AIDS, 4,* 901-907.

Healy, S. (1994). Diversity with a difference: On being old and lesbian. *Journal of Gay and Lesbian Social Services, 1,* 109-117.

Hellman, R. E., Stanton, M., Lee, J., Tytun, A., & Vachon, R. (1989). Treatment of homosexual alcoholics in government-funded agencies: Provider training and attitudes. *Hospital and Community Psychiatry, 40,* 1163-1168.

Helminiak, D. (1994). *What the Bible really says about homosexuality.* San Francisco, CA: Alamo Square Press.

Hemphill, E. (Ed.). (1991). *Brother to brother: New writings by black gay men.* Boston: Alyson.

Hencken, J. (1984). Conceptualizations of homosexual behavior which preclude homosexual self-labeling. *Journal of Homosexuality, 9*(4), 53-63.

Henry, G. (1948). *Sex variants: A study of homosexual patterns.* New York: Paul B. Hoeber.

Herdt, G. (1989). Gay and lesbian youth, emergent identities, and cultural scenes at home and abroad. *Journal of Homosexuality, 10*(1/2), 39-52.

Herdt, G., & Boxer, A. (1993). *Children of the horizons: How gay and lesbian teens are leading a new way out of the closet.* Boston: Beacon.

Herek, G. M. (1988). Heterosexuals' attitudes toward lesbians and gay men: Correlates and gender differences. *Journal of Sex Research, 25*(4), 451-477.

Herek, G. M. (1989). Hate crimes against lesbians and gay men: Issues for research and policy. *American Psychologist, 44*, 948-955.

Herek, G. M. (1992). The social context of hate crimes: Notes on cultural heterosexism. In G. Herek & K. Berrill (Eds.), *Hate crimes.* Thousand Oaks, CA: Sage.

Herek, G., & Berrill, K. (1992). *Hate crimes: Confronting violence against lesbians and gay men.* Newbury Park, CA: Sage.

Herek, G., & Glunt, E. (1988). An epidemic of stigma: Public reaction to AIDS. *American Psychologist, 43*, 886-891.

Herek, G., & Glunt, E. (1995). Identity and community among gay and bisexual men in the AIDS ear. In G. Herek & B. Greene (Eds.), *AIDS, identity, and community: The HIV epidemic and lesbians and gay men.* Thousand Oaks, CA: Sage.

Herschberger, S., & D'Augelli, A. R. (1995). The impact of victimization on the mental health and suicidality of lesbian, gay, and bisexual youths. *Developmental Psychology, 31*(1), 65-74.

Hetrick, E., & Martin, D. (1984). Ego dystonic homosexuality: A developmental view. In E. Hetrick & T. Stein (Eds.), *Innovations in psychotherapy with homosexuals.* Washington, DC: American Psychiatric Press.

Hickson, F., Davies, P. M., Hunt, A. J., Weatherburn, P., McManus, T. J., & Coxon, A. (1994). Gay men as victims of nonconsensual sex. *Archives of Sexual Behavior, 23*(3), 281-294.

Hitchcock, J., & Wilson, H. S. (1992). Personal risking: Lesbian self-disclosure of sexual orientation to professional health care providers. *Nursing Research, 41*, 178-183.

Hoeffer, B. (1981). Children's acquisition of sex-role behavior in lesbian mother families. *American Journal of Orthopsychiatry, 51*, 536-544.

Hooker, E. A. (1957). The adjustment of the male overt homosexual. *Journal of Projective Techniques, 21*, 17-31.

Hooker, E. A. (1967). The homosexual community. In J. Gagnon & W. Simon (Eds.), *Sexual deviance* (pp. 167-184). New York: Harper & Row.

Hudson, W., & Ricketts, W. (1980). A strategy for the measurement of homophobia. *Journal of Homosexuality, 5*, 357-371.

Huggins, S. L. (1989). A comparative study of self-esteem of adolescent children of divorced lesbian mothers and divorced heterosexual mothers. In

F. W. Bozett (Ed.), *Homosexuality and the family* (pp. 123-135). New York: Harrington Park Press.

Hunnisett, R. (1986). Developing phenomenological methods for researching lesbian existence. *Canadian Journal of Counseling, 20,* 255-286.

Hunter, J. (1994). Violence against lesbian and gay male youths. In G. Remafedi (Ed.), *Death by denial: Studies of suicide in gay and lesbian teenagers.* Boston: Alyson.

Icard, L., & Traunstein, D. M. (1987). Black, gay, alcoholic men: Their character and treatment. *Social Casework, 68,* 267-272.

Ireland, D., & Letellier, P. (1991). *Men who beat the men who love them: Battered gay men and domestic violence.* New York: Harrington Park Press.

Jenny, C., Roesler, T. A., & Poyer, K. L. (1994). Are children at risk for sexual abuse by homosexuals? *Pediatrics, 94*(1), 41-44.

Johnson, S. R., Guenther, S., Laube, D., & Keettel, W. (1981). Factors influencing lesbian gynecologic care: A preliminary study. *American Journal of Obstetrics and Gynecology, 140*(1), 20-28.

Johnson, S. R., & Palermo, J. (1984). Gynecologic care for the lesbian. *Clinical Obstetrics and Gynecology, 27,* 724-730.

Johnson, S. R., Smith, E. M., & Guenther, S. M. (1987a). Comparison of gynecologic health care problems between lesbians and bisexual women: A survey of 2,345 women. *Journal of Reproductive Health, 32,* 805-811.

Johnson, S. R., Smith, E. M., & Guenther, S. M. (1987b). Parenting desires among bisexual women and lesbians. *Journal of Reproductive Medicine, 32*(3), 198-200.

Johnston, M. A. (1992). A model program to address insensitive behaviors toward medical students. *Academic Medicine, 67*(4), 236-237.

Jones, C. (1978). *Understanding gay relatives and friends.* New York: Seabury Press.

Juzwiak, M. (1964, April). Understanding the homosexual patient. *RN, 27*(4), 53-59, 118.

Kahn, M. (1991). Factors affecting the coming out process for lesbians. *Journal of Homosexuality, 21*(3), 47-70.

Katz, J. N. (1982). *Gay/lesbian almanac: A new documentary.* New York: Harper & Row.

Katz, J. N. (1992). *Gay American history: Lesbians and gay men in the U.S.A.* (Rev. ed.). New York: Meridian.

Katz, J. N. (1995). *The invention of heterosexuality.* New York: Dutton.

Kavanagh, K., & Kennedy, P. (1992). *Promoting cultural diversity: Strategies for health care professionals.* Newbury Park, CA: Sage.

Kelly, J. A., St. Lawrence, J. S., Smith, S., Hood, H. V., & Cook, D. J. (1987). Medical students' attitudes towards AIDS and homosexual patients. *Journal of Medical Education, 62,* 549-556.

Kelly, J. A., St. Lawrence, J. S., Hood, H. V., Smith, S., & Cook, D. J. (1988). Nurses' attitudes toward AIDS. *Journal of Continuing Education in Nursing, 19,* 78-83.

Kimmel, D., & Sang, B. (1995). Lesbians and gay men in midlife. In A. D'Augelli & C. Patterson (Eds.), *Lesbian, gay, and bisexual identities over the lifespan: Psychological perspectives.* New York: Oxford.

Kinsey, A. C., Pomeroy, W. B., & Martin, C. E. (1948). *Sexual behavior in the human male.* Philadelphia: W. B. Saunders.

Kinsey, A. C., Pomeroy, W. B., Martin, C. E., & Gebhard, P. H. (1953). *Sexual behavior in the human female.* Philadelphia, PA: W.B. Saunders.

Kippax, S., Crawford, J., Connell, B., Dowsctt, G., Watson, L., Rodden, P., Baxterm, D., & Berg, R. (1992). The importance of gay community in the prevention of HIV transmission: A study of Australian men who have sex with men. In P. Aggleton, P. Davies, & G. Hart (Eds.), *AIDS: Rights, risks, and reason.* London: Falmer.

Kirkpatrick, M. (1989). Lesbians: A different middle age? In J. Oldham & R. Liebert (Eds.), *The middle years: New psychoanalytic perspectives.* New Haven, CT: Yale University Press.

Kirkpatrick, M., Smith, C., & Roy, R. (1981). Lesbian mothers and their children: A comparative study. *American Journal of Orthopsychiatry, 51,* 545-551.

Kitzinger, C. (1987). *The social construction of lesbianism.* London, England: Sage.

Klein, F., Sepekoff, B., & Wolf, T. J. (1985). Sexual orientation: A multi-variable dynamic process. *Journal of Homosexuality, 11*(1/2), 35-49.

Klepfisz, I. (1982). Anti-semitism in the lesbian/feminist movement. In E. T. Beck (Ed.), *Nice Jewish girls.* Watertown, MA: Persephone Press.

Klinkenberg, D., & Rose, S. (1994). Dating scripts of gay men and lesbians. *Journal of Homosexuality, 26*(4), 23-25.

Kooden, H., Morin, S., Riddle, D., Rogers, M., Sang, B., & Strassburger, F. (1979). *Removing the stigma: Final report of the Board of Social and Ethical Responsibility for Psychology's task force on the status of lesbian and gay male psychologists.* Washington, DC: American Psychological Association.

Koss, M. P. (1990). The women's mental health research agenda: Violence against women. *American Psychologist 45,* 374-380.

Kourany, R. F. (1987). Suicide among homosexual adolescents. *Journal of Homosexuality, 13*(4), 111-117.

Krafft-Ebing, R. von. (1886). *Psychopathia sexualis.* (G. Chaddock, Trans.). Philadelphia: F.A. Davis.

Kronemeyer, R. (1980). *Overcoming homosexuality.* New York: MacMillan.

Kurdek, L. A. (1988). Perceived social support in gays and lesbians in cohabitating relationships. *Journal of Personality and Social Psychology, 54,* 504-509.

Kurdek, L. A. (1994). The nature and correlates of relationship quality in gay, lesbian, and heterosexual cohabiting couples: A test of the individual, difference, interdependence, and discrepancy models. In B. Greene & G. Herek (Eds.), *Lesbian and gay psychology: Theory, research, and clinical applications* (pp. 133-155). Thousand Oaks, CA: Sage.

Kurdek, L. A. (1995). Lesbian and gay couples. In A. D'Augelli & C. Patterson (Eds.), *Lesbian, gay, and bisexual identities over the lifespan: Psychological perspectives.* New York: Oxford.

Kurdek, L. A., & Schmitt, J. (1986). Relationship quality of partners in heterosexual married, heterosexual cohabitating, and gay and lesbian relationships. *Journal of Personality and Social Psychology, 51,* 711-730.

Kus, R. J. (1995). *Addiction and recovery in gay and lesbian persons.* New York: Harrington Park Press.

Larsen, K., Reed, M., & Hoffman, S. (1980). Attitudes of heterosexuals toward homosexuality: A Likert type scale and construct validity. *Journal of Sex Research, 2,* 245-257.

Lassiter, S. (1995). *Multicultural clients: A professional handbook for health care providers and social workers.* Westport, CT: Greenwood Press.

LaTorre, R. A., & Wendenburg, K. (1983). Psychological characteristics of bisexual, heterosexual, and homosexual women. *Journal of Homosexuality, 9*(1), 87-97.

Lawrence, J. (1975). Homosexuals, hospitalization, and the nurse. *Nursing Forum, 14,* 305-317.

Leavy, R., & Adams, E. (1986). Feminism as a correlate of self-esteem, self-acceptance, and social support among lesbians. *Psychology of Women Quarterly, 10,* 321-326.

Lee, J. Y. (1996). Why Suzi Wong is not a lesbian. In B. Beemyn & M. J. Eliason (Eds.), *Queer studies: A lesbian, bisexual, gay, transgender reader.* New York: New York University Press.

Leigh, B. C. (1990). The relationship of substance use during sex to high risk sexual behavior. *Journal of Sex Research, 27,* 199-213.

Leininger, M. (1978). *Transcultural nursing: Concepts, theories, and practices.* New York: Wiley.

Leininger, M. (Ed.). (1991). *Culture care diversity and universality: A theory of nursing.* New York: National League for Nursing Press.

Lester, L., & Beard, B. (1988). Nursing students' attitudes toward AIDS. *Journal of Nursing Education, 27,* 399-404.

LeVay, S. (1991). A difference in hypothalamic structure between heterosexual and homosexual men. *Science, 253,* 1034-1037.

Levine, M. D., & Leonard, R. (1984). Discrimination against lesbians in the workforce. *Signs, 9,* 700-710.

Lim-Hing, S. (1994). *The very inside: An anthology of writing by Asian and Pacific Islander lesbian and bisexual women.* Toronto: Sister Vision.

Lohrenz, L. J., Connelly, J. C., Coyne, L., & Spare, K. E. (1978). Alcohol problems in several midwestern homosexual communities. *Journal of Studies on Alcohol, 39,* 1959-1963.

Loiacano, D. K. (1989). Gay identity issues among Black Americans: Racism, homophobia, and the need for validation. *Journal of Counseling and Development, 68,* 21-25.

Lorde, A. (1980). *The cancer journals.* San Francisco: Spinsters/Aunt Lute.

Lorde, A. (1982). *Zami: A new spelling of my name*. Freedom, CA: Crossing Press.

Loulan, J. (1984). *Lesbian sex*. San Francisco: Spinsters.

Loulan, J. (1987). *Lesbian passion: Loving ourselves and each other*. San Francisco, CA: Spinsters/Aunt Lute.

Lucas, V. (1992). An investigation of the health care preferences of the lesbian population. *Health Care for Women International, 13*(2), 221-228.

Lynch, J., & Reilly, M. (1985/1986). Role relationships: Lesbian perspectives. *Journal of Homosexuality, 12*, 53-69.

Lynch, M. A. (1993). When the patient is also a lesbian. *AWHONNS: Clinical Issues in Perinatal and Women's Health Nursing, 4*(2), 196-202.

MacDonald, A. P. (1976). Homophobia: Its roots and meaning. *Homosexual Counseling Journal, 3*, 23-33.

Malyon, A. K. (1982). Psychotherapeutic implications of internalized homophobia in gay men. *Journal of Homosexuality, 7*, 59-70.

Marmor, M., Weiss, L. R., Lyden, M., Weiss, S. H., Saxinger, W. C., Spira, T., & Feorina, P. (1986). Possible female-to-female transmission of HIV [Letter to the editor]. *Annals of Internal Medicine, 105*, 969.

Martin, A. (1993). *The lesbian and gay parenting handbook*. New York: HarperCollins.

Martin, D., & Lyon, P. (1972/1991). *Lesbian/Woman* (Rev. ed.). New York: Bantam Books.

Mason-John, V., & Khambatta, A. (1993). *Lesbians talk: Making Black waves*. London, England: Scarlet Press.

Masters, W. H., & Johnson, V. E. (1979). *Homosexuality in perspective*. Boston: Little, Brown.

Matthews, C., Booth, M., Turner, J., & Kessler, L. (1986). Physicians' attitudes toward homosexuality—Survey of a California county medical society. *Western Journal of Medicine, 144*(1), 106-110.

Mays, V. M., & Cochran, S. D. (1986, August). *The Black Lesbian Relationship Project: Relationship experiences and the perception of discrimination*. Paper presented at the 94th Annual Convention of the American Psychological Association, Washington, DC.

Mays, V. M., Cochran, S. D., & Rhue, S. (1993). The impact of perceived discrimination on the intimate relationships of black lesbians. *Journal of Homosexuality, 25*(4), 1-14.

McCandlish, B. (1987). Against all odds: Lesbian mother family dynamics. In F. W. Bozett (Ed.), *Gay and lesbian parents* (pp. 23-38). New York: Praeger.

McClure, M., & Vespry, A. (Eds.). (1994). *Lesbian health guide*. Toronto, Canada: Queer Press.

McDaniel, L. A. (1989). *Preservice adjustment of homosexual and heterosexual military accessions: Implications for security clearance suitability*. (PER-TR-89-004). Monterey, CA: Defense Personnel Security Research and Education Center.

McGhee, R. D., & Owen, W. F. (1980). Medical aspects of homosexuality. *New England Journal of Medicine, 303*(1), 50–51.

McKirnan, D. J., & Peterson, P. L. (1989a). Alcohol and drug use among homosexual men and women: Epidemiology and population characteristics. *Addictive Behaviors, 14,* 545–553.

McKirnan, D. J., & Peterson, P. L. (1989b). Psychosocial and cultural factors in alcohol and drug abuse: An analysis of a homosexual community. *Addictive Behaviors, 14,* 555–563.

McMichael, P. (1994). Toothpaste, socks, and contradictions. In J. Penelope (Ed.), *Out of the class closet: Lesbians speak.* Freedom, CA: Crossing Press.

McNaught, B. (1993). *Gay issues in the workplace.* New York: St. Martin's Press.

McWhirter, D., & Mattison, A. (1984). *The male couple: How relationships develop.* Englewood Cliffs, NJ: Prentice-Hall.

Meiselman, K. C. (1978). *Incest: A psychological study of causes and effects with treatment recommendations.* New York: Jossey-Bass.

Meisenhelder, J. B., & LaCharite, C. (1989). Fear of contagion: The public response to AIDS. *Image, 21*(1), 7–9.

Miller, B. (1979). Gay fathers and their children. *Family Coordinator, 28,* 544–552.

Minton, H., & McDonald, G. (1984). Homosexual identity formation as a development process. *Journal of Homosexuality, 9*(2/3), 91–104.

Miranda, J., & Storms, M. (1989). Psychological adjustments of lesbians and gay men. *Journal of Counseling and Development, 68,* 41–45.

Moberly, E. (1992, Fall). Can homosexuals *really* change? *Journal of Christian Nursing,* 14–17.

Molgaard, C. A., Nakamura, C., Hovell, M., & Elder, J. P. (1988). Assessing alcoholism as a risk factor for acquired immunodeficiency syndrome (AIDS). *Social Science and Medicine, 27,* 1147–1152.

Monzon, O. T., & Capellan, J. M. B. (1987). Female-to-female transmission of HIV. *The Lancet, 2*(8549), 40–41.

Morales, E. S. (1989). Ethnic minority families and minority gays and lesbians. *Marriage and Family Review, 14,* 217–239.

Morbidity and Mortality Weekly Report (1995, February 3). *Update: Acquired immunodeficiency syndrome—United States, 1994.* Atlanta: Centers for Disease Control.

Morgan, K. S. (1992). Caucasian lesbians' use of psychotherapy: A matter of attitude? *Psychology of Women Quarterly, 16,* 127–130.

Morgan, K. S., & Eliason, M. J. (1992). The role of psychotherapy in Caucasian lesbians' lives. *Women and Therapy, 13*(4), 27–52.

Morin, S. F. (1977). Heterosexual bias in psychological research on lesbianism and male homosexuality. *American Psychologist, 32,* 629–637.

Murphy, B. C. (1989). Lesbian couples and their parents: The effects of perceived parental attitudes on the couple. *Journal of Counseling and Development, 68,* 46–51.

Murphy, B. C. (1992). Educating mental health professionals about lesbian and gay issues. *Journal of Homosexuality, 22*(3/4), 229-246.

Murphy, T. F. (1992). Redirecting sexual orientation: Techniques and justifications. *Journal of Sex Research, 29*(4), 501-523.

Nardi, P. (1982). Alcoholism and homosexuality: A theoretical perspective. In D. J. Pittman & H. R. White (Eds.), *Society, culture, and drinking patterns reexamined* (pp. 285-305). New Brunswick, NJ: Rutgers Center for Alcohol Studies.

Nardi, P. (1991). Alcoholism and homosexuality: A theoretical perspective. In D. J. Pittman & H. R. White (Eds.), *Society, culture, and drinking patterns reexamined.* New Brunswick, NJ: Rutgers Center for Alcohol Studies.

Nardi, P. M., & Sherrod, D. (1994). Friendship in the lives of gay men and lesbians. *Journal of Social and Personal Relationships, 11,* 185-199.

Navratilova, M. (1993). Martina. In B. Singer (Ed.), *Growing up gay.* New York: New Press.

Neugarten, B., Wood, V., Kraines, R., & Loomis, B. (1963). Women's attitudes toward the menopause. *Vita Humana, 6,* 140-151.

Newman, B., & Muzzonigro, P. G. (1993). The effects of traditional family values on the coming out process of gay male adolescents. *Adolescence, 28*(109), 213-226.

Noyes, L. E. (1982). Gray and gay. *Journal of Gerontological Nursing, 11,* 636-639.

Nurius, P. A. (1983). Mental health implications of sexual orientation. *Journal of Sex Research, 19,* 119-136.

Oakley, A. (1993). *Essays on women, medicine, and health.* Edinburgh, Scotland: Edinburgh University Press.

O'Donnell, L., O'Donnell, C., Pleck, J., Snarey, J., & Rose, R. (1987). Psychosocial responses to hospital workers to Acquired Immune Deficiency Syndrome (AIDS). *Journal of Applied Social Psychology, 17*(3), 269-285.

Olsen, M. R. (1987). A study of gay and lesbian teachers. *Journal of Homosexuality, 13*(4), 73-81.

O'Neill, J. F., & Shalit, P. (1992). Health care of the gay male patient. *Primary Care, 19*(1), 191-201.

Ostrow, D. G., Beltran, E., & Joseph, J. (1994). Sexual behavior research on a cohort of gay men, 1984-1990: Can we predict how men will respond to interventions? *Archives of Sexual Behavior, 23,* 531-552.

Owlfeather, M. (1988). Children of grandmother moon. In W. Roscoe (Ed.), *Living the spirit: A gay American Indian anthology.* New York: St. Martin's Press.

"Pablo." (1993). In R. Lucczak (Ed.), *Eyes of desire: A deaf gay and lesbian reader* (pp. 39-42). Boston: Alyson.

Paroski, P. A. (1987). Health care delivery and the concerns of gay and lesbian adolescents. *Journal of Adolescent Health Care, 8,* 188-192.

Patterson, C. J. (1992). Children of lesbian and gay parents. *Child Development, 63,* 1025-1042.

Patterson, C. J. (1994). Children of the lesbian baby boom: Behavioral adjustment, self-concepts, and sex-role identity. In B. Greene & G. Herek (Eds.), *Lesbian and gay psychology: Theory, research, and clinical applications* (pp. 156-175). Thousand Oaks, CA: Sage.

Paul, J. P. (1986). *Growing up with a gay, lesbian, or bisexual parent.* Unpublished doctoral dissertation, University of California, Berkeley.

Pennington, S. (1987). Children of lesbian mothers. In F. W. Bozett (Ed.), *Gay and lesbian parents* (pp. 58-74). New York: Praeger.

Peplau, L. (1993). Lesbian and gay relationships. In L. Garnetts & D. Kimmel (Eds.), *Psychological perspectives on lesbian and gay male experiences.* New York: Columbia University Press.

Peretti, P. O., & Banks, D. (1984). Negative psychological variables of the incestuous daughter of father-daughter incest. *Child Psychiatry Quarterly, 17*(1-2), 15-20.

Perry, S., Jacobsberg, L., & Fogel, K. (1989). Orogenital transmission of human immunodeficiency virus. *Annals of Internal Medicine, 111,* 951.

Peters, D. K., & Cantrell, P. J. (1991). Factors distinguishing samples of lesbian and heterosexual women. *Journal of Homosexuality, 21*(4), 1-15.

Peterson, J. L. (1995). AIDS-related risks and same-sex behaviors among African American men. In G. Herek & B. Greene (Eds.), *AIDS, identity, and community.* Thousand Oaks, CA: Sage.

Pharr, S. (1988). *Homophobia: A weapon of sexism.* Inverness, CA: Chardon Press.

Phillips, G., & Over, R. (1992). Adult sexual orientation in relation to memories of childhood gender conforming and gender nonconforming behaviors. *Archives of Sexual Behavior, 21,* 543-558.

Phillips, G., & Over, R. (1995). Differences between heterosexual, bisexual, and lesbian women in recalled childhood experiences. *Archives of Sexual Behavior, 24,* 1-20.

Pies, C. (1985). *Considering parenthood.* San Francisco, CA: Spinsters.

Pillard, R. C. (1988). Sexual orientation and mental disorders. *Psychiatric Annals, 18,* 51-56.

Pillard, R. C., Poumadere, J., & Carretta, R. A. (1982). A family study of sexual orientation. *Archives of Sexual Behavior, 11*(6), 511-520.

Plummer, K. (1975). *Sexual stigma: An interactionist account.* London, England: Routledge.

Pollack, S., & Vaughn, J. (Eds.). (1987). *Politics of the heart: A lesbian parenting anthology.* Ithaca, NY: Firebrand Books.

Ponse, B. (1978). *Identities in the lesbian world: The social construction of self.* London: Greenwood.

Ponse, B. (1984). The problematic meanings of "lesbian." In J. D. Douglas (Ed.), *The Sociology of Deviance* (pp. 25-33). Boston: Allyn & Bacon.

Posin, R. (1991). Ripening. In B. Sang, J. Warshow, & A. Smith (Eds.), *Lesbians at midlife.* San Francisco: Spinsters.

Prieur, A. (1990). Norwegian gay men: Reasons for continued practice of unsafe sex. *AIDS Education and Prevention, 2,* 109-115.

Quam, J. K., & Whitford, G. S. (1992). Adaptation and age-related expectations of older gay and lesbian adults. *The Gerontologist, 32*(3), 367-374.

Ramos, J. (Ed.). (1994). *Companeras: Latina lesbian anthology.* New York: Routledge.

Rand, C., Graham, D. L., & Rawlings, E. (1982). Psychological health and factors the court seeks to control in lesbian mother custody trials. *Journal of Homosexuality, 8*(1), 27-39.

Randall, C. (1987). *Attitudes of BSN educators in a midwestern state toward lesbians.* Dubuque, IA: University of Dubuque College of Nursing.

Randall, C. (1989). Lesbian phobia among BSN educators: A survey. *Cassandra: Radical Nurses' Journal, 6,* 23-26.

Rankow, E. J. (1995). Lesbian health issues for the primary care provider. *Journal of Family Practice, 40*(5), 486-493.

Reagan, P. (1981). The interaction of health professionals and their lesbian clients. *Patient Counseling and Health Education, 3,* 21-25.

Remafedi, G. (1985). Adolescent homosexuality. *Clinical Pediatrics, 24*(9), 481-485.

Remafedi, G. (1994). Introduction: The state of knowledge on gay, lesbian, and bisexual youth suicide. In G. Remafedi (Ed.), *Death by denial: Studies of suicide in gay and lesbian teenagers.* Boston: Alyson.

Remafedi, G., Farrow, J. A., & Deisher, R. (1991). Risk factors for attempted suicide in gay and bisexual youth. *Pediatrics, 87*(6), 869-875.

Renzetti, C. M. (1989). Building a second closet: Third party responses to victims of lesbian partner abuse. *Family Relations, 38*(2), 157-163.

Renzetti, C. M. (1992). *Violent betrayal: Partner abuse in lesbian relationships.* Newbury Park, CA: Sage.

Rhoades, R. A. (1995). Learning from the coming-out experiences of college males. *Journal of College Student Development, 36*(1), 67-74.

Rich, C. L., Fowler, R. C., Young, D., & Blenkush, M. (1986). The San Diego suicide study: Comparison of gay to straight males. *Suicide and Life Threatening Behavior, 16,* 448-457.

Rich, J. D., Buck, A., Tuomala, R. E., & Kazanjian, P. H. (1993). Transmission of Human Immunodeficiency Virus infection presumed to have occurred via female homosexual contact. *Clinical Infectious Diseases, 17,* 1003-1005.

Ricketts, W., & Achtenberg, R. (1990). Adoption and foster parenting for lesbians and gay men: Creating new traditions in family. In F. W. Bozett & M. B. Sussman (Eds.), *Homosexuality and family relations* (pp. 83-118). New York: Harrington Park Press.

Riley, M. (1975). The avowed lesbian mother and her right to child custody: A constitutional challenge that can no longer be denied. *San Diego Law Review, 12,* 799-864.

Robertson, M. M. (1992). Lesbians as an invisible minority in the health services arena. *Health Care for Women International, 13*(2), 155-164.

Robertson, P., & Schachter, J. (1981). Failure to identify venereal disease in a lesbian population. *Sexually Transmitted Diseases, 8*(2), 75-76.

Robinson, B. E., & Skeen, P. (1982). Sex-role orientation of gay fathers versus gay nonfathers. *Perceptual and Motor Skills, 55,* 1055-1059.

Robinson, B. E., & Skeen, P., & Flake-Hudson, C. (1982). Sex role endorsement among homosexual men across the lifespan. *Archives of Sexual Behavior, 11*(4), 355-359.

Roesler, T., & Deisher, R. (1972). Youthful male homosexuality: Homosexual experience and the process of developing homosexual identity in males ages 16 to 22 years. *Journal of the American Medical Association, 219,* 1018-1023.

Rofes, E. (1995). Making our schools safe for sissies. In G. Unks (Ed.), *The gay teen: Educational practices and theory for lesbian, gay, and bisexual adolescents.* New York: Routledge.

Romo-Carmona, M. (1987). Introduction. In J. Ramos (Ed.), *Compañeras: Latina lesbians.* New York: Routledge.

Roscoe, W. (1987). Bibliography of berdache and alternative gender roles among North American Indians. *Journal of Homosexuality, 14,* 81-171.

Rose, P. (1993). Out in the open? Lesbianism. *Nursing Times, 89*(30), 50-52.

Rose, P., & Platzer, S. (1993). Confronting prejudice: Gay and lesbian issues. *Nursing Times, 89*(31), 52-54.

Rosser, S. V. (1993). Ignored, overlooked, or subsumed: Research on lesbian health and health care. *National Womens' Studies Association Journal, 5*(2), 183-203.

Rothblum, E. (1990). Depression among lesbians: An invisible and unresearchable phenomenon. *Journal of Gay and Lesbian Psychotherapy, 1*(3), 67-87.

Rothblum, E. (1994). "I only read about myself on the bathroom walls": The need for research on the mental health of lesbians and gay men. *Journal of Consulting and Clinical Psychology, 62*(2), 213-220.

Ruefli, T., Yu, D., & Barton, J. (1992). Sexual risk taking in smaller cities: The case of Buffalo, NY. *Journal of Sex Research, 29,* 95-108.

Rust, P. (1992). The politics of sexual identity: Sexual attraction and behavior among lesbian and bisexual women. *Social Problems, 39,* 366-386.

Rust, P. (1993). "Coming out" in the age for social constructionism. *Gender and Society, 7,* 50-77.

Rust, P. (1996). Sexual identity in the social landscape. In B. Beemyn & M. J. Eliason (Eds.), *Queer studies: A lesbian, gay, bisexual and transgender reader.* New York: New York University Press.

Sabatini, M., Patel, K., & Hirschman, R. (1984). Kaposi's sarcoma and T-cell lymphoma in an immunodeficient woman: A case report. *AIDS Research, 1,* 135-137.

Saghir, M. T., & Robins, E. (1973). *Male and female homosexuality: A comprehensive investigation.* Baltimore: Williams and Wilkins.

Saghir, M. T., Robins, E., Walbran, B., & Gentry, K. A. (1970a). Homosexuality III: Psychiatric disorders and disability in the male homosexual. *American Journal of Psychiatry, 126,* 1079-1086.

Saghir, M. T., Robins, E., Walbran, B., & Gentry, K. A. (1970b). Homosexuality IV: Psychiatric disorders and disability in the female homosexual. *American Journal of Psychiatry, 127,* 147-154.

Saint, A. (1991). Hooked for life. In E. Hemphill (Ed.), *Brother to brother: New writings by black gay men* (pp. 136-141). Boston: Alyson.

Sandfort, T. G. M. (1995). HIV/AIDS prevention and the impact of attitudes toward homosexuality and bisexuality. In G. Herek & B. Greene (Eds.), *AIDS, identity, and community: The HIV epidemic and lesbians and gay men.* Thousand Oaks, CA: Sage.

Sang, B. (1991). Moving toward balance and Integration. In B. Sang, J. Warshaw, & A. Smith (Eds.), *Lesbians at midlife: The creative transition.* San Francisco, CA: Spinsters.

Saunders, J. M., Tupac, J., & McCullouch, B. (1988). *A lesbian profile: A survey of 1000 lesbians.* West Hollywood, CA: Southern California Women for Understanding.

Saunders, J. M., & Valente, S. M. (1987). Suicide risk among gay men and lesbians: A review. *Death Studies, 11*(1), 1-23.

Savin-Williams, R. C. (1989). Coming out to parents and self-esteem among gay and lesbian youths. *Journal of Homosexuality, 20*(3/4), 27-87.

Savin-Williams, R. C. (1994). Verbal and physical abuse as stressors in the lives of lesbian, gay male and bisexual youths: Associations with school problems, running away, substance abuse, prostitution, and suicide. *Journal of Consulting and Clinical Psychology, 62*(2), 261-269.

Scherer, Y., Haughey, B., & Wu, Y. (1989). AIDS: What are nurses' concerns? *Clinical Nurse Specialist, 3,* 48-54.

Schilit, R., Clark, W. M., & Shallenberger, E. A. (1988). Social supports and lesbian alcoholics. *Women and Social Work, 3*(2), 27-40.

Schilit, R., Lie, G. Y., & Montagne, M. (1990). Substance use as a correlate of violence in intimate lesbian relationships. *Journal of Homosexuality, 19*(3), 51-65.

Schmidt, G., & Clement, U. (1995). Does peace prevent homosexuality? *Journal of Homosexuality, 28,* 269-276.

Schmitt, J. P., & Kurdek, L. A. (1987). Personality correlates of positive identity and relationship involvement in gay men. *Journal of Homosexuality, 13*(4), 101-109.

Schwanberg, S. L. (1990). Attitudes toward homosexuality in American health care literature 1983-1987. *Journal of Homosexuality, 19*(3), 117-136.

Scroggs, R. (1983). *Homosexuality in the New Testament: Contextual background for contemporary debate.* Philadelphia: Fortress Press.

Sears, J. T. (1989). The impact of gender and race on growing up lesbian and gay in the South. *National Women's Studies Association Journal, 1,* 422-457.

Sedgwick, E. (1990). *Epistemology of the closet.* Berkeley, CA: University of California Press.

Sell, R. L., Wells, J. A., Valleron, A. J., Will, A., Cohen, M., & Umbel, K. (1990, June). *Homosexual and bisexual behavior in the United States, the United*

Kingdom and France. Paper presented at the Sixth International Conference on AIDS, San Francisco, CA.

Shidlo, A. (1994). Internalized homophobia: Conceptual and empirical issues in measurement. In B. Greene & G. Herek (Eds.), *Lesbian and gay psychology: Theory, research, and clinical applications* (pp. 176-205). Thousand Oaks, CA: Sage.

Siever, M. D. (1994). Sexual orientation and gender as factors in socioculturally acquired vulnerability to body dissatisfaction and eating disorder. *Journal of Consulting and Clinical Psychology, 62*(1), 252-260.

Silvera, M. (1990). Man royals and sodomites: Some thoughts on the invisibility of Afro-Caribbean lesbians. In S. D. Stone (Ed.), *Lesbians in Canada.* Toronto, Canada: Between the Lines.

Silvera, M. (Ed.). (1991). *Piece of my heart: A lesbian of colour anthology.* Toronto, Canada: Sister Vision Press.

Silverstein, C. (1991). Psychological and medical treatments of homosexuality. In J. Gonsiorak & J. Weinrich (Eds.), *Homosexuality: Research implications for public policy.* Newbury Park, CA: Sage.

Simari, C. G., & Baskin, D. (1982). Incestuous experiences within homosexual populations: A preliminary study. *Archives of Sexual Behavior, 11*(4), 329-343.

Skinner, W. F. (1994). The prevalence and demographic predictors of illicit and licit drug use among lesbians and gay men. *American Journal of Public Health, 84*(8), 1307-1310.

Slater, S. (1995). *The lesbian family life cycle.* New York: Free Press.

Slocum, M. (1993). A united front. In B. Hunter (Ed.), *Sojourner: Black gay voices in the age of AIDS.* New York: Other Countries.

Smith, E. M., Johnson, S. R., & Guenther, S. M. (1985). Health care attitudes and experiences during gynecologic care among lesbians and bisexuals. *American Journal of Public Health, 75*(9), 1085-1087.

Socarides, C. W. (1975). *Beyond sexual freedom.* New York: Quadrangle.

Sophie, J. (1985/1986). A critical examination of stage theories of lesbian identity development. *Journal of Homosexuality, 12,* 39-51.

Spector, R. (1991). *Cultural diversity in health and illness.* Norwalk, CT: Appleton & Lange.

Stall, R., & Wiley, J. (1988). A comparison of alcohol and drug use patterns of homosexual and heterosexual men: The San Francisco Men's Health Study. *Drug and Alcohol Dependence, 22,* 63-73.

Steckel, A. (1985). *Separation-individuation in children of lesbian and heterosexual couples.* Unpublished doctoral dissertation, Wright Institute Graduate School, Berkeley, CA.

Steckel, A. (1987). Psychosocial development of children of lesbian mothers. In F. W. Bozett (Ed.), *Gay and lesbian parents* (pp. 75-85). New York: Praeger.

Stephany, T. M. (1992). Faculty support for gay and lesbian nursing students. *Nurse Educator, 17*(5), 22-23.

Stephany, T. M. (1993). Lesbian hospice patients. *Home Healthcare Nurse, 11*(6), 65.

Stevens, P. (1992). Lesbian health care research: A review of the literature from 1970-1990. In P. Stern (Ed.), *Lesbian health: What are the issues?* Washington, DC: Taylor and Francis.

Stevens, P. (1993a). Lesbians and HIV: Clinical, research, and policy issues. *American Journal of Orthopsychiatry, 63,* 289-294.

Stevens, P. (1993b). Marginalized women's access to health care: A feminist analysis. *Advanced Nursing Science, 16*(2), 39-56.

Stevens, P. (1994). Protective strategies of lesbian clients in home health care environments. *Research in Nursing and Health, 17,* 217-229.

Stevens, P., & Hall, J. (1988). Stigma, health beliefs, and experiences with health care in lesbian women. *IMAGE, 20,* 69-73.

Stine, G. (1995). *AIDS update, 1994-95.* Englewood Cliffs, NJ: Prentice-Hall.

Strommen, E. F. (1989). "You're a what?": Family members' reactions to the disclosure of homosexuality. *Journal of Homosexuality, 18,* 37-58.

Terry, J. (1990). Lesbians under the medical gaze: Scientists search for remarkable differences. *Journal of Sex Research, 27*(3), 317-339.

Thompson, B. W. (1994). *A hunger so wide and so deep.* Minneapolis, MN: University of Minnesota Press.

Thompson, K., & Andrzejewski, J. (1988). *Why can't Sharon Kowalski come home?* San Francisco, CA: Spinsters/Aunt Lute Press.

Tremble, B., Schneider, M., & Apparthurai, C. (1989). Growing up gay or lesbian in a multicultural context. *Journal of Homosexuality, 17*(1-4), 253-267.

Triandis, H. C. (1982, August). *Incongruence between intentions and behavior: A review.* Paper presented at the American Psychological Association convention, Washington, DC.

Trippet, S. E. (1994). Lesbians' mental health concerns. *Health Care for Women International, 15,* 317-323.

Trippet, S. E., & Bain, J. (1990). Preliminary study of lesbian health concerns. *Health Values, 14*(6), 30-36.

Trippet, S. E., & Bain, J. (1993). Physical health problems and concerns of lesbians. *Women and Health, 20,* 59-70.

Troiden, R. (1988). *Gay and lesbian identity.* New York: General Hall.

Troll, L. (1989). *Continuations: Adult development and aging.* Baltimore: University of Maryland International University Consortium.

Turner, R. K., Pielmaier, H., James, S., & Orwin, A. (1974). Personality characteristics of male homosexuals referred for aversion therapy: A comparative study. *British Journal of Psychiatry, 125,* 447-449.

Turque, B. (1992, September 14). Gays under fire. *Newsweek,* 35-40.

U.S. Departments of Agriculture and Health and Human Services (1987). *Cross-cultural counseling: A guide for nutrition and health counselors.* Washington, DC: Author.

Vasquez-Pacheco, R. (1993). Necropolis. In B. M. Hunter (Ed.), *Sojourner: Black gay voices in the age of AIDS.* New York: Other Countries Press.

Vincke, J., Bolton, R., Mak, R., & Blank, S. (1993). Coming out and AIDS-related high risk sexual behavior. *Archives of Sexual Behavior, 22,* 559-586.

von Schulthess, B. (1992). Violence in the streets: Anti-lesbian assault and harassment in San Francisco. In G. Herek & K. Berrill (Eds.), *Hate crimes.* Thousand Oaks, CA: Sage.

Wallick, M., Cambre, K., & Townsend, M. (1992). How the topic of homosexuality is taught at U.S. medical schools. *Academic Medicine, 67*(9), 601-603.

Warren, N. (1993, October/November). Out of the question: Obstacles to research on HIV and women who engage in sexual behavior with women. *SIECUS Report, 22*(1), 13-16.

Waterman, C. K., Dawson, L. J., & Bologna, M. J. (1989). Sexual coercion in gay male and lesbian relationships: Predictors and implications for support services. *Journal of Sex Research, 26,* 118-124.

Weinberg, G. (1972). *Society and the healthy homosexual.* New York: St. Martin's Press.

Weinberg, M. S., & Bell, S. (1972). *Homosexuality: An annotated bibliography.* New York: Harper & Row.

Weinberg, M. S., & Williams, C. J. (1974). *Male homosexuals: Their problems and adaptations.* New York: Oxford University Press.

Weinberg, M. S., Williams, C. J., & Pryor, D. W. (1994). *Dual attractions: Understanding bisexuality.* New York: Oxford University Press.

Weinberg, T. S. (1978). On "doing" and "being" gay: Sexual behaviors and homosexual male self-identity. *Journal of Homosexuality, 4*(2), 143-156.

Weinberg, T. S. (1994). *Gay men, drinking and alcoholism.* Carbondale, IL: Southern Illinois University Press.

Wells, J. W., & Kline, W. B. (1987). Self-disclosure of homosexual orientation. *Journal of Social Psychology, 127,* 191-197.

Wells, R. J. (1987). AIDS—A perspective of care. *International Nursing Review, 34*(3), 64-66.

West, C. (1993). *Race matters.* Boston: Beacon Press.

Weston, K. (1991). *Families we choose: Lesbians, gays, and kinship.* New York: Columbia University Press.

WHCoA helps coalesce policy agenda on gay/lesbian aging. (1995). *Aging Today,* September/October, p. 10.

Whitman, F. L. (1977). Childhood indicators of male homosexuality. *Archives of Sexual Behavior, 6,* 89-96.

Whitman, F. L., Diamond, M., & Martin, J. (1993). Homosexual orientation in twins: A report on 61 pairs and three triplet sets. *Archives of Sexual Behavior, 22*(3), 187-205.

White, E. (Ed.). (1990). *Black women's health book: Speaking for ourselves at last.* Seattle, WA: Seal Press.

White, T. A. (1979). Attitudes of psychiatric nurses toward same sex orientations. *Nursing Research, 28*(5), 276-281.

Wicker, A. W. (1969). Attitudes versus actions: The relationship of verbal and overt behavioral respondes to attitude objects. *Journal of Social Issues, 25,* 41-78.

Wilson, G. D. (1987). Male-female differences in sexual activity, enjoyment and fantasies. *Personality and Individual Difference, 8,* 125-127.

Winnow, J. (1989/1990, Winter). Lesbians evolving health care: Our lives depend on it. *Sinister Wisdom, 39,* 33-62.

Wismont, J. M., & Reame, N. E. (1989). The lesbian childbearing experience: Assessing developmental tasks. *IMAGE: Journal of Nursing Scholarship, 21*(3), 137-141.

Young, E. W. (1988). Nurses' attitudes toward homosexuality: Analysis of change in AIDS workshops. *Journal of Continuing Education in Nursing, 19*(1), 9-12.

Young, M. (1992, Fall). Leaving the lesbian lifestyle. *Journal of Christian Nursing, 9*(4), 11-13.

Zeidenstein, L. (1990). Gynecological and childbearing needs of lesbians. *Journal of Nurse-Midwifery, 35,* 10-18.

Zuger, B. (1984). Early effeminate behavior in boys: Outcome and significance for homosexuality. *Journal of Nervous and Mental Disease, 172*(2), 90-97.

Index

Acceptance:
  parental, 85, 143
  significance of, 28, 228
Accessibility, to health care, 5
ACT-UP, 55
Adolescent homosexuality:
  coming out process, 142–143
  depression, 143
  HIV, 144
  homelessness, 144
  implications of, 20, 85, 105
  parents of, working with,
    146–147
  pregnancy, 144
  prostitution, 144
  sexual identity development,
    139–142
  sexually transmitted infections,
    144
  suicide, 143
  violence and, 143–144
  working with, guidelines for,
    145–146
Adoption, 82–83, 99–100, 173
African Americans:
  discrimination experiences, 150
  stereotypes, 34, 36
Ageist stereotypes, 156
Aging process, 152–153, 157
AIDS, see HIV/AIDS
  in adolescents, 144

AIDS in real life exercise, 210
education programs, 222
in gay/bisexual men, 203–209
health care provider attitudes,
    111, 114, 117–119
homosexual incidence of, 12
social support, 94
stigmatization, 207
transmission:
  fears, 117–118
  female-to-female, 167
  stereotypes, 77–79
in women:
  etiology, 167–168
  lack of information, 169–170
  reactions to, 168–169
Alcohol abuse:
  by gay/bisexual men, 195–198
  by lesbian/bisexual women, 170,
    175–178
Alcoholics Anonymous (AA), 180
American Academy of Pediatrics,
    147
American Association of Physicians
    for Human Rights (AAPHR),
    224
Amyl nitrate, 198
Anal cancer, 201
Androgyny, 68–69
Anorexia, 183
Anti-Semitism, 54

Anxiety, social, 44
Asian Americans:
  racism, 49
  stereotypes, 36
AT&T, 221
Attitudes:
  acceptance, 28
  celebration, 27-28
  disapproval, 29
  disgust, 29
  hatred, 30-31
  of health care providers, *see*
    Health care providers,
    attitudes
  negative, *see* Negative attitudes
  societal, 81-83
  tolerance, 28-29
Attitude toward Homosexuality Scale
  (ATHS), 112-113
Aversion therapy, 24

Bem Sex-Role Inventory, 115
Berdache, 50
Bible interpretations, 53, 63-67
Biologically-based sexual
  orientation, 56-58
Bio-psycho-social-cultural sexuality
  model, 57
Biphobia, 79, 162
Bisexuality:
  stereotypes, 78-79
  in women, 40
Blended families, 100
Bottoms, Sharon, 81, 96
Bowie, David, 69
Boyhood Gender Conformity Scale,
  133
Brabant, Joe, 159
Bulimia, 183

Cancer:
  in gay men, 201
  in lesbian/bisexual women,
    170-171
Candidiasis, vaginal, 166-167

Career/work issues, 150-151. *See
  also* Discrimination, employee;
  Employee benefits
Celebration attitude, 27-28
Celibacy, 26
Censorship, 6
Center for Disease Control (CDC),
  167-168
Center for Epidemiologic Studies
  Depression Scale (CES-D), 182
Cervical dysplasia, 167
Cervicitis, 166
Childhood:
  play activities, 68
  sexual identity development,
    131-139
Child molestation stereotypes,
  70-71
Children, of same-sex relationships:
  coming out to, 100-102
  gender identity, 96
  gender role behavior, 96
  objections to, 95-96
  other-sex role models, 98-100
  peer relations, 97-98
  personality development, 97
  sexual orientation, 97
  societal attitudes and, 81-83
  statistics, 83
  unique problems of, 102
Chlamydia, 166
Christian doctrine, 66
Churches, antigay teaching, 6
Cigarette smoking, 170-171
Civil rights laws, 4
Clinical training, 219
Cognitive therapy, 77
Coming out process:
  in adolescence, 142-143
  case illustration, 84-85
  cycles of, 41-43
  defined, 32, 37
  economic model of, 44-45
  family, disclosure to, 83-86,
    142-143

health care providers, disclosure to, 91–92, 119–128
identity formation, 38–44
in middle adulthood, 154
parenting guidelines, 86
in young adulthood, 148–149
Commitment:
  by health care institutions, 223–224
  in same-sex relationships:
    significance of, 88
    in young adulthood, 149–150
Communication skills, health care providers:
  interviewing techniques, 184–186
  overview, 226–228
  terminology, 26, 88–89
Communities, homosexual:
  age factors, 53
  gender differences, 51–52
  historical perspective, 19
  political involvement, 54–55
  racial and ethnic diversity in, 45–51
  religious diversity, 53–54
  socioeconomic classes, 52–53
Compartmentalization, 157
Confrontational health care providers, 179
Co-parents, rights of, 102
Coping skills, 105
Criminal attacks, 19–20, 30, 45, 93, 143–144. See also Gay-bashing; Rape; Sexual assault
Cross-gender behavior, 138
Cultural diversity, 3
Cultural homophobia, 31, 33. See also Heterosexism
Cures, historical perspective, 23–24
Custody cases, 81–82, 99, 104
Cystic breast disease, 170

Dating surveys, 149
Defense mechanisms, 33, 148, 226

Depression:
  in gay/bisexual men, 192–194
  implications of, 20–21, 33, 44, 105, 143
  in lesbian/bisexual women, 181–182
Developmental transitions:
  adolescence, 139–147
  childhood, 131–139
  middle adulthood, 151–155
  older adulthood, 155–160
  young adulthood, 147–151
Diagnostic and Statistical Manual of Mental Disorders (DSM), 21–22, 138
Disability, 94
Disapproval, 29
Disclosure, to health care providers, 91–92, 119–128, 164. See also Coming out process
Discrimination:
  case illustrations, 42, 150
  employee, 220–221
  racial, see specific races
Disgust, 29
Disney World, 221
Domestic violence, 33, 94, 180, 194–195
Donor insemination (DI), 100, 104, 172–173
Drug abuse:
  by gay/bisexual men, 198–200
  by lesbian/bisexual women, 177–178, 180–181
Drug therapies, 23–24

Eating disorders, 182–183
ECT (electroconvulsive therapy), 29
Egodystonic homosexuality, 21
Elders, Jocelyn, Surgeon General, 35
Elder services, 158–160
Ellis, Albert, 18
Embarrassment, 43, 101
Empathy training, 31
Employee benefits, 222

Empty nest syndrome, 153
Environmentally-based sexual
     orientation, 58
Erikson, Erik, 149
Estrogen, 77
Estrus cycle, 57
Etheridge, Melissa, 69
Ethics codes, 228-229
European Americans:
     racism, 46-47
     stereotypes, 36
Exodus International, 186

Family issues:
     children of same-sex couples,
          95-103
     coming out process, see Coming
          out process
     family of origin, 83-87
     "family values" exercise, 105-106
     gay/lesbian families, 87-95
     health care providers strategies,
          103-105
Family Law, significant events in,
     99
Family of origin, 83-87
Family practice physicians, goals
     for, 226
Family relationships:
     coming out process, 44, 83-84,
          142-143
     homophobia and, 32
Family values exercise, 105-106
Fears, types of, 43, 119, 189
Flaunting sexuality stereotypes, 73,
     75
Freedman, Marcia, 159
Freud, Sigmund, 18

Gay bars, 19, 30, 197
Gay-bashing, 93, 143, 189-192
Gay Community News, 119
Gay ghettos, 22
Gay liberation movement, 21-22
Gay organizations, 22-23

Gay pride events, 55
Gender, defined, 25
Gender benders, 26
Gender differences:
     aging process, 152-153, 158
     childhood play activities, 68, 132
     coming out process, 86-87
     in gay communities, generally,
          51-52
     gender nonconformity, 132, 139
     health issues, see Men's health;
          Women's health
     in midlife, 152-155
     in relationships, 87-88
     suicide rates, 143
     violence, 94
Gender identity, 26
Gender identity disorder, 132, 138
Gender nonconformity research,
     132-139
Generativity, 151
Genital herpes, 166-167
Gonorrhea, 166
Guardianship, 9
Guilt:
     coming out process, 43, 83-85
     gender nonconforming behavior,
          139
     internalized homophobia, 33
Gynecological care, 164-166

Hagman, Larry, 78
Hate crimes:
     against men, 189-192
     against women, 183-184
Hatred, 30-31
Health care education, 109
Health care institutions, changes
     needed in:
     climate, 214-215
     education and training, 216-220
     overview, 214-216, 225
     patient policies, 224-225
     policies and procedures, 220-224
     social atmosphere, 215-216

Health care literature, 110-111, 216-217
Health care providers:
  adolescents, working with, 145-146
  antigay violence, dealing with, 93-94
  attitudes:
    AIDS and homosexuality, 117-119, 204-207
    negative, 123-129, 163
    survey of, 112-116
    types of, 109-112
  changes needed in, 229-225
  communication skills, 226-228
  experiences dealing with:
    health care perceptions, 121-128
    sexual identity disclosure, 119-121
  family relationships, strategies for dealing with, 103-105
  interaction styles, 179-180
  sexual identity disclosure to, 91-92, 119-121, 164, 227
Health care system:
  research needs, 231-232
  self-protective strategies for dealing with, 127-128
Health issues, mental and physical, see Men's health; Women's health
Heterosexism, 5, 33-37
Heterosexual aversion, 24, 70
Heterosexuals Attitudes toward Homosexuality Scale (HATH), 113-114
HIV/AIDS:
  in gay/bisexual men, 203-209
  health care provider attitudes, 204-207
  historical overview, 203
  in lesbian/bisexual women, 166-170
  prevention of, 207-209

social support, 94
stereotypes, 78
transmission, female-to-female, 167
Homelessness, 144
Homeopathic remedies, 129, 165
Homophobia:
  in adolescents, 141
  AIDS phobia and, 119
  attitudes toward, 27-30
  as a continuum, 31
  cultural, 31
  defined, 5, 27, 162
  elimination of, 212-213
  family life and, 102
  gender differences, 113
  health care provider roles, 103-105
  historical perspective, 27
  implications of, 2, 32
  Index of, 59-61
  institutional, 31
  internalized, 32-33, 41, 72, 79, 91, 93, 99, 141, 192-200, 208
  interpersonal, 31
  manifestations of, 128
  racism and, 47
Homosexuality:
  historical overview, 18-24
  population statistics, 11-13
  terminology, 24-26
Hospice care, 228
Hospitalization, 95, 211
Human papilloma virus, 165-167
Human sexuality, education and training, 218-220
Hypothalamus, 57

Identity:
  exploration, 41-42
  formation, stages of, 38-44
  gender, 26
  reevaluation, 42
  sexual, see Sexual identity
Illness, 94
Incest, 70, 171

Index of Homophobia, 59-61
Influential health care providers, 179
Institutional homophobia, 31
Internalized homophobia, implications of, 32-33, 41, 72, 79, 91, 93, 99, 141, 192-200, 208
Internalized racism, 42
Interpersonal homophobia, 31
Interracial relationships, 47
Interstitial nuclei of the anterior hypothalamus (INAH3), 57
Invalidation experiences, 42

Jackson, Michael, 69
Jagger, Mick, 69
John, Elton, 69
Jokes, antigay, 5
Judeo-Christian doctrine, 53-54

King James, 34
Kinsey Report, 11-12
Kochman, Arlene, 159
Kowalski, Sharon, 7-10, 91-92

lang, k. d., 69
Latinos, racism and, 48-49
Lawrence of Arabia, 35
Lesbian baby boom, 83
Lesbian & Gay Aging Issues Network (LGAIN), 159
Lesbianism:
    vs. gay men, see Gender differences
    gender roles and, 68-69
    racism and, 48-50
    sexual reorientation treatments, 76-77
Levi Strauss, 223
Lifestyle, defined, 26
Little Richard, 69
Lockheed, 223

Mantle, Mickey, 78
Marital status, 34

Marriage, as "cure," 86
Masturbation, 35, 75
Maternalistic health care providers, 179
Media, antigay concerns, 6, 34, 39, 139
Menopause, 153-155
Men's health:
    mental:
        depression, 192-194
        domestic violence, 194-195
        hate crimes, 189-192
        internalized homophobia, potential consequences of, 192-200
        substance abuse, 195-200
        suicide, 192-194
    physical:
        HIV/AIDS, 203-209
        unsafe sexual experiences, 200-202
Menstruation, 141-142. See also Menopause
Metropolitan Church of Christ, 66
Michelangelo, 35
Microsoft, 221
Middle adulthood, in homosexuals:
    implications of, 53, 151-153
    male issues, 154-155
    reproductive transitions, 153-154
Midlife crises, 153, 156
Minorities, internalized homophobia and, 193-194
Modern homosexual, 23

National health care, 211
Native Americans:
    racism and, 50
    stereotypes, 36
Negative attitudes:
    in health care literature, 110-111
    in health care providers, 123, 127-129, 163
    implications of, 4, 6, 22, 33

Negative stereotypes:
  AIDS transmission, 77-78
  Bible interpretations, 63-67
  bisexuality, 78-79
  child molestation, 70-71
  early sexual experiences and,
    69-70, 74
  flaunting sexuality, 73, 75
  implications of, generally, 62-63,
    80
  promiscuity, 71-72
  sex obsession, 72-73
  sexual inverts, 67-69
  sexual preferences, 75-77
Nondiscrimination policy:
  employment issues, 221
  sexual orientation and, 103-104,
    221
North American Man-Boy Love
  Association (NAMBLA), 71

Oedipal complex, 58
Older adulthood, homosexual:
  elder services, 158-160
  implications of, 53, 155-158
  planning for, 160
Open marriage, 86
"Open secret," 85
Opposite sex, 25
Overeating, compulsive, 183

Pap smear, 164-165
Parades, 55
Parental acceptance, 85, 143
Parental influence:
  maternal knowledge of sexual
    identity, 135-136
  sexual orientation and, 58, 84. See
    also Children, of same-sex
    relationships
Parenting:
  adolescent homosexuals and,
    146-147
  routes to, 100, 172-173
Paternalistic health care providers,
  179

Pedophiles, 71
Pelvic inflammatory disease,
  166-167
Personality traits, stereotyping, 68
PFLAG (Parents and Friends of
  Lesbians and Gays), 85, 146
Physical attraction, 51
Political involvement, 54-55
"Poppers," 198
Pornography, 195
Post-traumatic Stress Disorder, 93
Pregnancy, 144, 172-173
Preidentity, 41
Prejudice:
  defined, 5
  global, 3-4
  implications of, 6-7
  learning, 5-6
  types of, generally, 111
Prince, 69
Procter & Gamble, 221
Proctitis, 201
Promiscuity, 71-72
Prostitution, 144
Psychoanalytic theory, sexual
  orientation, 84
Psychological tests, 20-21

Queer Nation, 55

Racial identity, 42, 46
Racism, 5, 42, 46-48
Rape, 69, 171, 190-191, 194-195
Reaction formation, 148
Receptive anal sex (RAS), 209
Relationships, same-sex:
  characteristics of, 88-89
  with children, see Children, of
    same-sex relationships
  conflict sources, 91
  dissolution of, 91
  formation of:
    generally, 72, 89
    in young adulthood, 149-150
  hospitalization, 95
  illness/disability issues, 94

Relationships, same-sex *(Continued)*
  satisfaction in, 87, 89–90, 155
  sexually exclusive, 89–90
  social support, 87–88
  stages in, 90
  violence and, 92–94
Religious beliefs, impact of, 29–31,
    53–54
Reparative therapies, 22–23, 75–77
Role models, 5, 233
Role-playing, 219, 226
Roosevelt, Eleanor, 35

Safe sex campaigns, 73
Safe sex practices, 169–170, 209
Sage, 159
SageNet, 159
Self-awareness, 148
Self-blame, 85, 93
Self-care, 129, 165
Self-confidence, 148
Self-definition, 143, 157
Self-destructive behavior, 41
Self-esteem, 43, 105, 139
Self-hatred, 33, 91
Self-labeling, 48
Sensitization, 24
Sex, defined, 25
Sex education, 33–35, 144, 169, 202,
    209
Sex hormones, sexual orientation:
  biologically-based research
      studies, 57, 77
  "redirecting" treatments, 76–77
Sexism, 5
Sex obsession, 72–73
Sexual abuse, implications of, 58,
    70–71
Sexual assault, 93, 190–191
Sexual attraction, 51
Sexual confusion, 148
Sexual dysfunctions, 171–172
Sexual experiences, early, 69–70, 74
Sexual identity:
  "confused" stereotype, 67–69
  defined, 25–26

determination exercise, 14–16
developmental transitions, *see*
    Developmental transitions
Sexual inverts, 67–69
Sexually exclusive relationships,
    89–90
Sexually transmitted infections
    (STIs), 144, 166
Sexual orientation:
  in children of same-sex
      relationships, 97
  defined, 25
  origin/"causes" of, 55–58
  "redirecting" treatments,
      75–76
Sexual preferences, 25, 75–77
Shame, 33, 43, 101, 105, 139
Siblings, disclosure to, 85–86
Significant other, terminology for,
    88–89
Social anxiety, 44
Social support, 87–88, 104
Societal attitudes, health care system
    and, 212–214
Socioeconomic class, 52–53
Sodomy laws, 104
Stereotypes:
  cultural, 3, 34, 36
  defined, 62
  distorted, 35–36
  exploration activity, 80
  health care provider research,
      115
  implications of, 62–63, 80
  negative, *see* Negative stereotypes
  personality traits, 68
Stigmatization, 11–12, 97, 138, 142
Stress reduction techniques, 105
Substance abuse:
  by gay/bisexual men, 195–200
  implications of, 21, 33, 41, 105,
      148
  by lesbian/bisexual women,
      175–181
Suicide attempts:
  by gay/bisexual men, 192–194

by lesbian/bisexual women,
181-182
statistics, 20-21, 33, 105, 143
Support groups, 223
Support systems, 87-88, 104
Surgical treatment, historical
perspective, 23
Syphilis, 166

Teenage homosexuals, *see*
Adolescent homosexuality
Testosterone, 76
Time/Warner, 223
Tolerance, 28-29
Tomboy behavior, 132, 134
Transgendered people, 26
Transsexuals, 26
Trichomonias, 166
Twin studies, sexual orientation
research, 56

US West, 221

Vaginal yeast infections, 166
Vaginitis, 166
Victim blaming, 93
Victimization:
in adolescence, 143-144
antigay violence, 93
women and, 183-184
Violence:
anti-gay, 93-94, 143, 189-192
same-sex couples and, 92-94. *See
also* Domestic violence
Visitation rights, case illustration,
7-11
Voyeurism, 127, 227

White, Dan, 190
White, Mel, 54

White House Conference on Aging
(WHCOA), 159-160
Whitman, Walt, 35
Women's health:
interviewing techniques, 184-186
mental:
depression, 181-182
eating disorders, 182-183
generally, 173-175
hate crimes, 183-184
substance abuse/misuse,
175-181
suicide attempts, 181-182
physical:
cancers, 170-171
generally, 163-164
gynecological care, 164-166
HIV/AIDS, 166-170
lack of information on,
161-163
pregnancy-related issues,
172-173
sexual dysfunctions, 171-172
sexually transmitted infections
(STIs), 166
Women's liberation movement, 21
Work setting, inclusive organization
exercise, 187
Worthlessness, feelings of, 93

X chromosome, 56
Xerox, 221

Young adulthood:
career/work issues, 150-151
coming out process, 148-149
commitment, to partner/family,
50
intimate relationships, forming,
149-150